Disc	Root	Motor	Sensory	Reflex
C5-C6	C6	Biceps, wrist ext.	Med. arm & hand	Biceps
C6-C7[1]	C7	Triceps, wrist flex.	Middle finger	Triceps
C7-T1	C8	Finger flex.	Lat. hand	Finger
L3-L4	L4	Quadriceps	Med. calf	Knee
L4-L5[1]	L5	Dorsiflexors	Med. foot	
L5-S1	S1	Plantar flexors	Lat. foot	Ankle

Table 1. Symptoms of disc herniation. [1] Most common.

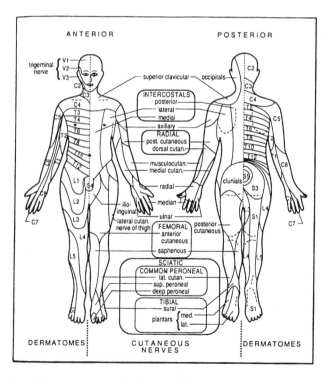

Figure 2. Dermatomes and peripheral nerve territories. (From Patton HD, et al. *Introduction to Basic Neurology.* Philadelphia: WB Saunders, 1976, with permission.)

ACKNOWLEDGEMENTS

I want to thank my witty, tolerant editor, Charley Mitchell at Lippincott Williams and Wilkins. Many colleagues at MGH and other institutions have helped me immeasurably by reading portions of the text, or by influencing the way I think. They include Drs. Robert Brown, Ferdinando Buonanno, Apostolos Caneris, Keith Chiappa, Andrew Cole, Michael Cutrer, Merit Cudkowicz, Clifford Eskey, Steven Greenberg, Michael Greene, John Growdon, Samuel Hahn, John Henson, John Herman, Daniel Hoch, David Hooper, J. Philip Kistler, Barry Kosofsky, C. J. Malanga, Stephen Parker, John Penney, Jonathan Rosand, Jeremy Schmahmann, Lee Schwamm, Marion Stein, Katharina Trede, and especially Shirley Wray. Any remaining errors are my fault, not theirs. Anne Young, Walter Koroshetz, and Andrew Hrycyna deserve several paragraphs of individual thanks, but this is a tiny book, so they only get a sentence.

This book is dedicated to Jack (John B.) Penney, Professor of Neurology at Harvard, Neurologist at MGH, and Director of the MIT-MGH Parkinson's Disease Center. He died suddenly on January 31, 1999, at the age of 51. None of us can believe it yet. He leaves behind his wife, Anne B. Young, daughters Jessica and Ellen, a heartsick department and laboratory, bereft patients, former trainees throughout the country, and the many families with Huntington's disease on Lake Maracaibo, Venezuela, whom he visited yearly for the past 18 years.

FRONT COVER
Functional MRI evidence that even the simplest "See A, do B" algorithms of this handbook require brain activation. The cover shows images of a retinotopic map during a visual task (medial view), and of the hand map during a sensorimotor task (lateral view). The images were provided by Janine Mendola and Christopher Moore of the MGH NMR Center.

THE MASSACHUSETTS GENERAL HOSPITAL

HANDBOOK OF NEUROLOGY

Alice Flaherty, M.D., Ph.D.
Massachusetts General Hospital
Harvard Medical School
Boston, Massachusetts

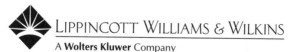

LIPPINCOTT WILLIAMS & WILKINS
A **Wolters Kluwer** Company

Philadelphia · Baltimore · New York · London
Buenos Aires · Hong Kong · Sydney · Tokyo

Acquisitions Editor: Charles W. Mitchell
Developmental Editor: Raymond E. Reter
Production Editor: Robert Pancotti
Manufacturing Manager: Kevin Watt
Cover Designer: Diana Andrews
Printer: R. R. Donnelley, Crawfordsville

© 2000 by LIPPINCOTT WILLIAMS & WILKINS
227 East Washington Square
Philadelphia, PA 19106-3780 USA
LWW.com

Printed in the USA

Library of Congress Cataloging-in-Publication Data

Flaherty, Alice.
 The Massachusetts General Hospital handbook of neurology/Alice Flaherty.
  p. ;cm.
Includes bibliographical references and index.
ISBN 0-683-30576-X
 1. Neurology—Handbooks, manuals, etc. 2. Nervous system—Diseases—Handbooks, manuals, etc. 3. Medical protocols. I. Title: Handbook of neurology. II. Massachusetts General Hospital. III. Title.
 [DNLM: 1. Nervous System Diseases—Handbooks. 2. Neurology—Handbooks. WL 39 F575m 2000]
RC355 .F56 2000
616.8—dc21

                                                                              99-045312

Care has been taken to confirm the accuracy of the information presented and to describe generally accepted practices. However, the author and publisher are not responsible for errors or omissions or for any consequences from application of the information in this book and make no warranty, expressed or implied, with respect to the currency, completeness, or accuracy of the contents of the publication. Application of this information in a particular situation remains the professional responsibility of the practitioner. "Be careful about reading health books. You may die of a misprint"—Mark Twain.

The author and publisher have exerted every effort to ensure that drug selection and dosage set forth in this text are in accordance with current recommendations and practice at the time of publication. However, in view of ongoing research, changes in government regulations, and the constant flow of information relating to drug therapy and drug reactions, the reader is urged to check the package insert for each drug for any change in indications and dosage and for added warnings and precautions. This is particularly important when the recommended agent is a new or infrequently employed drug.

Some drugs and medical devices presented in this publication have Food and Drug Administration (FDA) clearance for limited use in restricted research settings. It is the responsibility of the health care provider to ascertain the FDA status of each drug or device planned for use in their clinical practice.

10 9 8 7 6 5 4 3 2 1

CONTENTS

FOREWORD

This handbook has been used for the past several years at the Massachusetts General Hospital, Brigham and Women's Hospital, and West Roxbury V. A. Hospital. It is aimed at housestaff, fellows, and other hospital-based practitioners. It is not a primer; its intent is to remind busy clinicians of what they should already know. Nonetheless, the medical students and nurses on our service have also found it useful, as have housestaff in internal medicine, neurosurgery, and psychiatry. Despite the many neurology handbooks available, Alice Flaherty had the energy, drive, and dedication to develop her own because she knew we needed:

An up-to-date, algorithmic approach. The protocols presented here include recent changes, such as thrombolysis. They are in keeping with current medical trends towards developing specific, uniform approaches to diagnosis and management. Algorithms are, of course, intended as an adjunct to thought, not a replacement for it. They should not be applied blindly.

An emphasis on efficient diagnosis and treatment. Medical and surgical management techniques are described in detail. Dr. Flaherty has chosen to give specific recommendations, realizing that there may be other equally valid approaches.

Coverage of modern imaging techniques, such as diffusion-weighted MRI. Many other neurology texts are still organized around neuropathology, not neuroradiology. This results in problems such as brainstem diagrams that are presented in the pathological rather than radiological convention. To help interpret an MRI, such diagrams must be mentally rotated 180° in two planes - no easy feat when you are reading a scan emergently at 4 am.

Integration of allied disciplines. The current trend away from subspecialization makes it imperative that neurologists be able to recognize and manage common medical, neurosurgical and psychiatric problems. Alice Flaherty includes concise sections on these issues, as well as a mini-pharmacopoeia, so that clinicians need not carry more than one manual.

Anne B. Young, M.D., Ph.D.
Chief of Neurology, Massachusetts General Hospital
Julieanne Dorn Professor of Neurology, Harvard Medical School

ABBREVIATIONS

Abbreviations used only locally are defined in that section.

A fib	atrial fibrillation
Ab	antibody
Abx	antibiotics
ABG	acute blood gas
ACA	anterior cerebral artery
ACE	angiotensin-converting enzyme
ACE-I	ACE inhibitor
A-comm	anterior communicating artery
ACTH	adrenocorticotropic hormone
ADHD	attention-deficit hyperactivity disorder
AFB	acid-fast bacillus stain for TB
Ag	antigen
AICA	anterior inferior cerebellar artery
AKA	also known as
ALS	amyotrophic lateral sclerosis
ANA	antinuclear antibody
ANS	autonomic nervous system
AV	atrioventricular
AVM	arteriovenous malformation
BBB	bundle branch block
bid	twice a day
BP	blood pressure
BUN	blood urea nitrogen
Ca	calcium
CAD	coronary artery disease
CBC	complete blood count
CHF	congestive heart failure
Cl	chloride
CMV	cytomegalovirus
CN	cranial nerve
CNS	central nervous system
COPD	chronic obstructive pulmonary disease
CPAP	continuous positive airway pressure
CPK	creatine phosphokinase
Cr	creatinine
CSF	cerebrospinal fluid
CT	computed tomograph
CXR	chest X-ray
CZI	crystallinezine insulin
D5	5% dextrose
DBP	diastolic blood pressure
DDAVP	vasopressin
DDx	differential diagnosis
DIC	disseminated intravascular coagulation
DM	diabetes mellitus
DTR	deep tendon reflex
DVT	deep venous thrombosis
DWI	diffusion-weighted MRI
dz	disease
EBV	Epstein-Barr virus
EEG	electroencephalogram
EKG	electrocardiogram
EMG	electromyography
EOM	extraocular movement
ER	emergency room
ESR	erythrocyte sedimentation rate
ETT	exercise tolerance test

GABA	gamma-aminobutyric acid
GBM	glioblastoma multiformae
GBS	Guillain-Barré syndrome
GI	gastrointestinal
H&P	history and physical exam
h/o	history of
HA	headache
HCG	human chorionic gonadotrophin
Hct	hematocrit
Hg	mercury
HLA	human leukocyte group A
HOB	head of bed
HR	heart rate
HSV	herpes simplex virus
HTN	hypertension
I/Os	inputs and outputs
ICA	internal carotid artery
ICH	intracranial hemorrhage
ICP	intracranial pressure
ICU	intensive care unit
Ig	immunoglobulin
IM	intramuscular
INR	international normalized PTT ratio
IQ	intelligence quotient
IU	international units
IV	intravenous
IVDA	intravenous drug abuse
K	potassium level
L	left
LAD	left anterior descending artery
LFT	liver function test
LMN	lower motor neuron
LOC	loss of consciousness
LP	lumbar puncture
LV	left ventricle
MAOI	monoamine oxidase inhibitor
Max.	maximum
MCA	middle cerebral artery
MCV	mean corpuscular volume
MI	myocardial infarction
MRA	magnetic resonance angiogram
MRI	magnetic resonance image
MS	multiple sclerosis
N/V	nausea and vomiting
NCS	nerve conduction studies
NG	nasogastric tube
nl	normal
NPH	normal pressure hydrocephalus
NPO	nothing by mouth
NS	normal saline
NSAID	nonsteroidal antiinflammatory drug
nu.	nucleus
OR	operating room
PCA	posterior cerebral artery
P-comm	posterior communicating artery
PCR	polymerase chain reaction
PE	pulmonary embolus
PET	positron emission tomography
PICA	posterior inferior cerebellar artery

PMN	polymorphonuclear leukocyte	SIADH	syndrome of inappropriate antidiuretic hormone secretion
PNS	peripheral nervous system		
PO	by mouth	SIEP	serum immunoelectrophoresis
PPD	purified protein derivative test for TB	SL	sublingual
		SLE	systemic lupus erythematosus
PR	per rectum	SPECT	single-photon emission computed tomography
Pre-op	preoperative		
prn	as needed	SQ	subcutaneous
PSNS	parasympathetic nervous system	SRI	serotonin reuptake inhibitor
pt	patient	Sx	symptoms, signs
PT	prothrombin time	TB	tuberculosis
PTT	partial thromboplastin time	TCA	tricyclic antidepressant
PTX	pneumothorax	TEE	transesophageal echocardiogram
q	Latin: *quaque* (every)	TIA	transient ischemic attack
qd	daily	TIBC	total iron-binding content
qhs	nightly	tid	three times a day
qid	four times a day	TSH	thyroid stimulating hormone
qod	every other day	UA	urinalysis
QTc	QT interval, corrected for HR	UBJ	urine Bence-Jones protein
R	right	UMN	upper motor neuron
r/o	rule out	US	ultrasound
RBC	red blood cell	V fib	ventricular fibrillation
REM	rapid eye movement sleep	V tach	ventricular tachycardia
RF	rheumatoid factor	V/Q	ventilation-perfusion lung scan
RPR	rapid plasmin reagent test	VDRL	venereal disease research laboratory test
RV	right ventricle		
Rx	treatment	VP	ventriculoperitoneal
SAH	subarachnoid hemorrhage	VS	vital signs
SBP	systolic blood pressure	VZV	varicella zoster virus
SC	subcutaneous	WBC	white blood cell
SCA	superior cerebellar artery	XRT	radiation therapy
SDH	subdural hemorrhage		

EMERGENCIES

ADMISSIONS

The most critical parts of the exam are underlined.

GENERAL EXAM

A. VS: <u>BP, HR, temperature</u>, respirations, orthostatic BP.
B. Skin: Petechiae, rash, striae, telangiectasias, caput medusae.
C. Head: For trauma exam, see p. 89.
    1. Eye: <u>Papilledema</u>, retinopathy, icterus.
    2. Skull: Trauma, craniotomy.
    3. Other: Temporal wasting or tenderness, ears, nose, throat.
D. Neck: <u>Stiffness, carotids/bruits</u>, thyroid, jugular distension, nodes.
E. Back: <u>Lungs</u>, spine tenderness, pelvic stability.
F. Chest: <u>Heart</u>, breasts, nodes.
G. Abdomen: Bowel sounds, bruits, palpation, nodes, liver, hernias, scars.
H. Genitourinary: Hair, testis size/masses, lesions, pelvic exam.
I. Rectal: <u>Guaiac</u>, masses, tenderness, tone.
J. Limbs: <u>Pulses</u>, color, edema, splinters/clubbing, calf pain, Homan's sign, range of motion, straight leg raise.

NEUROLOGICAL EXAM

A. Mental status: For coma exam, see p. 24. For psychiatric mental status exam (including the Mini-Mental Status Exam), see p. 76.
    1. Orientation: <u>Date, place</u>.
    2. Attention: <u>Say months backwards</u>; spell "world" backwards.
    3. Memory: <u>3 objects, presidents</u>.
    4. Speech: <u>Naming, fluency, comprehension, repetition,</u> reading, writing.
        a. F test: Number of words beginning with F in 60 sec (nl >12 if high school education).
        b. Comprehension of passive constructions.
    5. Frontal:
        a. Perseveration: Go-no go task, copying Luriia diagram.
        b. Disinhibition: Snout, grasp, imitation behavior.
        c. Abulia: Affect, response latency.
    6. Parietal:
        a. Neglect: <u>Limb recognition,</u> clock draw, bisect line.
        b. Calculations: Serial 7's, etc.
        c. Praxis: Orobuccal apraxia is often L hemisphere lesion; dressing apraxia often R.
        d. Spatial orientation: Directions, commands across midline.
        e. Agnosia: Finger agnosia, anosagnosia, alexia without agraphia, color naming.
    7. Cognition: Insight, judgement, proverbs, similes, subjunctives, logic.
    8. Thought content: Paranoia, ideas of reference, delusions, hallucinations.
    9. Mood: SIGECAPS criteria, suicidal or homicidal ideation, mania.
B. Cranial nerves:

I: Smell.

II: <u>Pupils, fundi; fields</u>, acuity, blink to threat, red desaturation. Pts. with hysterical (or cortical) blindness will have normal pupils, blink to threat.

III, IV, VI: <u>Horner's syndrome, EOMs</u>, saccades, pursuit, optokinetic reflex, cover-uncover test, red glass test, upper lid.

V: <u>Sensation</u> of forehead/cheek/chin, corneals, jaw.

VII: <u>Symmetry</u>, brow raise, eye close, nose wrinkle, grimace, cheek puff, anterior taste.

VIII: Tympani, hearing (see p. 45), Bárány's test.

IX, X, XI, XII: <u>Palate, tongue</u>, gag, sternocleidomastoid, trapezius.

C. Motor:
1. **Strength:** <u>Drift, fine finger movements, heel/toe walk, knee bends.</u>
   a. **Individual muscles:** Include hip adductors, pronation/supination, inversion/eversion, abdominal muscles.
   b. **Subtle signs:** Wortenberg's (pull flexed fingers; thumb flexes), stress gait (walk on outside of feet, look for posturing), mirror movements with finger sequencing, testing multiple repeats.
   c. **Hysteria:**
      1) **"Give-way" weakness:** May see jerky relaxation in weak limb when test both limbs together (can also see this with poor proprioception).
      2) **Hoover's sign:** Have pt. lie down, hold your hand under the normal heel while pt. raises the weak leg against resistance. In hysterical weakness, the pt. does not push down into your hand with the normal leg, whereas he or she will if the weakness is real.
2. **Bulk:** Atrophy, fasciculations.
3. **Tone:** Rigidity, spasticity, cogwheeling, dystonic posturing, myotonia. If pt. not cooperative, drop limb to test tone (malingering pts. may not let limb hit face).
4. **Tremor:** Myoclonus, asterixis, intention tremor, chorea.
5. **Reflexes:** <u>Biceps, triceps, brachioradialis, knee, ankle, Babinski.</u>
   a. **If brisk:** Check clonus, spreading, palmomental, jaw jerk, Hoffman's sign (flick nail down, watch for thumb contraction).
   b. **If frontal damage:** Grasp, snout, suck.
   c. **If spinal cord injury:** Abdominals, suprapubic, cremasteric, wink, bulbocavernosus.

D. Cerebellar
1. **Appendicular:** <u>Finger-to-nose</u>, rapid alternating movements, fine finger movements, finger following, lack of check, toe tapping, heel-to-shin, decreased tone, arm swings after shaking shoulders (nl < 3), pendular reflexes.
2. **Axial:** <u>Gait, tandem gait</u>, stand on line, walk in circle, march with eyes close (advancing more than a few feet or rotating more 30 degrees in 30 sec. is abnormal).
3. **Voice:** Dysarthria, holding a tone, la-la-la, saying "Methodist-Episcopal," count to 20 fast.

E. Sensory:
1. **Pin:** <u>All 4 limbs</u>; trunk for level; nerve distributions, summation.

   a. Hysteria: See if numbness stops at hairline, or ask pt. when they feel it and see if they say "no" reliably each time you touch them.
2. **Light touch:** Cotton wisp; 2-point discrimination.
3. **Proprioception:** <u>Joint position, vibration, Romberg</u>, nose touch.
   a. Hysteria: See if vibration felt more strongly on one side of forehead than the other.
4. **Cortical:** <u>Double simultaneous extinction</u>, stereognosis, graphesthesia.
5. **Temperature**. Use side of tuning fork or alcohol swab.
6. **Anal:** If you suspect spinal cord lesion, check anal wink, tone, bulbocavernosus reflex.

ADMISSION ORDERS

A. **Notifications:** You may need to speak to the senior resident; private neurologist; internist, floor or nurse accepting the patient, or family members.
B. **Orders:** <u>ADCVAANDISCL</u>.
   1. **A**dmit: List service, admitting physician, resident to page.
   2. **D**iagnosis: Be specific.
   3. **C**ondition: Good, fair, guarded, critical.
   4. **V**ital signs: Specify if other than per routine.
   5. **A**llergies: List the reaction too, e.g. "contrast dye → anaphylaxis."
   6. **A**ctivity: Bedrest with HOB up 30 degrees? Out of bed with assist? Ad lib?
   7. **N**ursing: Pneumoboots? Guaiac all stools? Etc.
   8. **D**iet: NPO? Aspiration precautions? Low salt or cholesterol? Diabetic? Renal? Dysphagic?
   9. **I**ns/Outs: Done automatically in most ICUs; harder to do on general wards. If it is important, consider inserting a bladder catheter. Daily weights also are difficult on some floors and may take special urging.
   10. **S**pecial:
       a. **Oxygen or ventilator settings.**
       b. **Bleed risk?** Blood bank sample, guaiac stools, orthostatic BP, large-bore IV.
       c. **CHF?** Strict I/Os, daily weights.
       d. **Chest pain?** Oxygen, cardiac monitor, bedside commode, CPKs q8h x 3.
       e. **Mental status change?** (See p. 33) Restraint x 72 h prn safety, aspiration precautions.
       f. **Clot risk?** Pneumoboots, SC heparin, (if DVT, elevate foot, bedrest), neurovascular checks.
       g. **Hyper- or hypotension:** BP parameters and drugs.
       h. **Skin care**.
   11. **C**onsults: Consider social service, physical therapy, occupational therapy, speech,....
   12. **L**abs: bid PTT? Daily PT/INR? qod electrolytes/BUN/Cr?
C. **Drugs:** Consider
   1. **D5 NS** at 60 if concern for brain edema.
   2. **Bowel?** e.g. bisacodyl 1 tab PR qd prn, milk of magnesia 30 ml q8h prn.

3. **Sleeping pill?** See p.84. <u>Not</u> if pt. confused. Diphenhydramine 25-50 mg qhs prn), or lorazepam (0.5-1.0 mg).

4. **Pain?** Acetaminophen 650 mg q4h prn, or oxycodone 1-2 mg q4 prn, meperidine 50-100mg with hydroxyzine 25 mg q4h IM prn, slow-release morphine 10-30 mg q8h, etc.

5. **GI?** Aluminum and magnesium hydroxide 30ml q4h prn (if renal failure use only aluminum hydroxide). Consider sucralfate 1g qid, omeprazole 20 qd, ranitidine 150 bid (avoid if pt. on anticonvulsants).

6. **Diabetes?** NPH insulin + regular (CZI) sliding scale: for blood glucose < 200, 0U; 200-249, 2U; 250-299, 4U; 300-349, 6U; 350-399, 8U; > 400, 10U.

   a. **Hypertension?** e.g. nifedipine 10 mg PO q4h or metoprolol 50 mg PO bid prn SBP > 180. For IV drugs, see p. 136.

   b. **Hypotension?** IV fluids; consider midodrine 10 mg PO tid, or IV drugs (p. 136).

7. **Chest pain?** Avoid hypotension in stroke or carotid dz.

   a. **SL nitroglycerine:** 0.3 mg q5min prn x 3 while SBP > 120.

   b. **NTP SS:** q4h for SBP < 120, wipe; 120-134, 0.5 in.; 135-149, 1 in.; 150-164, 1.5 in.; > 165, 2 in.

D. Admission note: Chief complaint, history of present illness, past medical history, allergies, medicines, family and social history (always include education), review of systems, physical exam, labs, assessment, plan.

1. **Assessment by issues:** CNS, cardiovascular (pump, rate, rhythm, valves...), pulmonary, renal, fluids/electrolytes/nutrition, infectious dz, GI, GU, hematologic, endocrine, dermatologic, oncologic, orthopedic, psychiatric, rheumatologic, code status, discharge plan.

2. **Etiologies:** <u>TIM P, DIVE IN</u>. <u>T</u>raumatic/Toxic, <u>I</u>CP, <u>M</u>etabolic, <u>P</u>sychiatric, <u>D</u>egenerative/Deficiency, <u>I</u>nfectious, <u>V</u>ascular, <u>E</u>pileptic, <u>I</u>nflammatory, <u>N</u>eoplastic.

ADULT NEUROLOGY

APHASIA, AGNOSIA, APRAXIA, AND AMNESIA

A. Aphasia: Disordered language production; in distinction to the motor disability of dysarthria. Ask three questions: Is the patient's speech fluent? Does he comprehend speech? Can he repeat it?

Type of aphasia	Fluent?	Compre-hends?	Repeats?	Lesion
Global	No	No	No	Doesn't localize
Broca's (productive)	No	Yes	No	Inf. frontal gyrus
Wernicke's (receptive)	Yes	No	No	Sup. temporal gyrus
Transcortical motor	No	Yes	Yes	Premotor cortex
Transcortical sensory	Yes	No	Yes	Occipitotemporal cortex
Conductive	Yes	Yes	No	Subcortical MCA territ.
Amnestic (anomia)	Yes	Yes	Yes	Alzheimer's dz, etc.

Table 2. Major aphasia categories.

B. Evolution of aphasia: Broca's and Wernicke's aphasia from strokes commonly start as global aphasia acutely and only later become clearly productive or receptive aphasia. The amnestic aphasia of Alzheimer's dz may evolve into a full-blown Wernicke's aphasia.
C. Alexia, agraphia, and acalculia: Respectively, inability to read, write, and do arithmetic. Usually from lesions of the left angular gyrus. For alexia without agraphia, see Vision, p. 37.
D. Amnesia: Poor memory storage (anterograde amnesia) or recall (retrograde amnesia). Often from hippocampal or paramedian thalamic lesion.
E. Agnosia: Impairment of recognition in a single modality, as opposed to amnesia, in which impairment includes all modalities.
    1. Anosognosia: Unawareness of neurological deficit. Usually from right parietotemporal lesion.
    2. Neglect: Disregard of stimuli arising from one side of the body, usually the left, from right parietal lesion.
    3. Object agnosia: Usually from bilateral posterior temporal lobe lesion.
    4. Visual agnosias: See p. 38.
F. Apraxia: Inability to do a task for cognitive rather than motor reasons.
    1. Ideomotor apraxia: Disordered sequence of complex movement, e.g. by perseveration or distortion. From left premotor or parietal lesion.
    2. Constructional apraxia: Disorder of spatial design or drawing. From parietal lesion.

BRAINSTEM ANATOMY

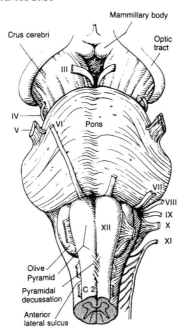

Figure 3. The ventral surface of the brainstem. (From Duus P. *Topical Diagnosis in Neurology.* New York: Thieme, 1983:101, with permission.)

A. See also: Cranial nerves, p. 27.
B. Slice anatomy: The following five images are in radiologic convention, as if looking up from the feet. This is upside-down and backwards from the neuropathological convention. In order, they show the midbrain, upper pons, mid-pons, lower pons, and upper medulla.

ANTERIOR
RIGHT ←|→ LEFT
POSTERIOR

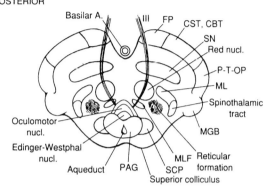

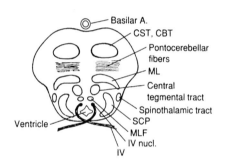

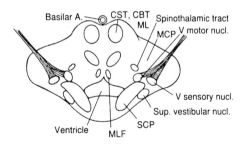

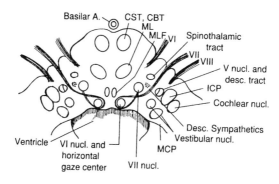

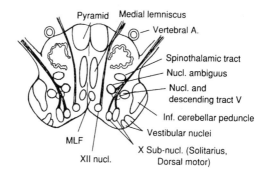

Figure 4. The brainstem in cross-section. (From Schwamm L. In Batjer HH, ed. *Cerebrovascular Disease*, Philadelphia: Lippincott-Raven, 1997:347-375, with permission).

CEREBROSPINAL FLUID

A. **Lumbar puncture:** See Procedures, p. 191.
B. **Diseases by CSF profile:**
   1. **Many PMNs, low sugar, high protein:**
      a. **Infectious:** Bacterial meningitis, early viral or TB meningitis, parameningeal infections, septic emboli.
      b. **Noninfectious:** Chemical meningitis, Behçet's dz, Mollaret's recurrent meningitis.
   2. **Many lymphocytes, low sugar, high protein:** TB, fungal, or partially treated/resolving bacterial meningitis, viral meningitis, leptomeningeal metastases.
   3. **Many lymphocytes, normal sugar, high protein:** Viral meningitis or encephalitis, partially treated/resolving bacterial meningitis, parameningeal infections, early fungal or TB meningitis, parasitic infections, postinfectious encephalomyelitis, active demyelinating dz.

C. CSF findings by disease:

Condition	OP (cm H$_2$O)	Color	Cells/mm^3	Protein (mg%)	Glucose (CSF÷Serum)	Miscellaneous
Normal adult	6-20	Colorless	0 PMN or RBC, <5 mono	15-45	0.5	Lymph/PMN ratio = 100/0
Normal child	6-20	Colorless	<5 WBCs	5-40	~0.5	
Normal term	8-10	Colorless	<8 WBCs	90	~0.5	Lym/PMN=40/60
Normal premie		Colorless	<9 WBCs	115	~0.5	Lym/PMN=40/60
Acute meningitis	nl or up	Turbid	>100 WBCs, mostly PMNs	100-1000	< 0.2	+ rapid antigen tests
Viral meningo-encephalitis	nl	nl	10-350 WBCs, mostly monos	40-100	nl	PMNs early
Guillain-Barré syndrome	nl	nl	nl to 100 monos	50-1000	nl	Protein nl early
Tuberculous meningitis	nl or up	Opal; clots on standing	50-500 lymphs and monos	60-700	0.2-0.4	+ AFB culture and stain
Fungal meningitis	nl or up	Opal	30-300 monos (PMNs early)	100-700	<0.3	+ India ink prep
HSV encephalitis	nl or up	Bloody	High monos and RBCs	High (nl early)	nl or low	nl WBCs in 3% PCR for antigen
Parameningeal infection	Up if block	nl	0-800 WBCs	High	nl	E.g. Epidural abscess
Traumatic (bloody) tap	nl	Bloody, no xantho.	RBC/WBC ratio like blood	Slightly up	nl	Blood less in following tubes
Subarachnoid hemorrhage	Up	Bloody, + xantho	RBC/WBC < blood; nl early	50-800	nl	RBCs last 2 wk; xantho longer
Multiple sclerosis	nl	nl	5-50 monos	nl-800	nl	Oligoclonal igG
Neurosyphilis	nl	nl	0-300	High (nl late)	nl	Oligoclonal igG, treponema Ab
Leptomeningeal metastasis	nl or up	Usually nl	0-500	nl or up	nl	Cytology shows tumor in 50%
Pseudotumor cerebri	25-50	nl	nl	nl	nl	Do large-volume therapeutic tap
Toxoplasmosis	nl or up	nl	nl or up	Usu. Hi	~nl	CSF often nl

Table 3. CSF findings by disease.

D. Skull CSF leak

1. **H&P:** Skull trauma, nasal or ear drainage when leaning forward or sneezing. Have pt. lean forward for several minutes to elicit nasal discharge.
2. **Labs:** To show if nasal fluid is CSF (rather than snot): glucose > 20, chloride > serum Cl. Tau transferrin.
3. **Rx:** Lumbar drain; prophylactic nafcillin x 3 days. Hang bag as low as possible without causing headache (usually level of heart).

E. LP headache or spinal CSF leak: See Headache, p. 43.

CEREBROVASCULAR ISCHEMIA

A. **Acute stroke:** Treat as an emergency if thrombolysis is an option, if sx are fluctuating (especially if correlated with BP), if it is a large cerebellar stroke, or if there are signs of herniation.
B. **See also:** Venous sinus thrombosis, p. 98, Transient monocular blindness, p. 35, Hemorrhagic infarcts, p. 52.

C. H&P: Symptom onset, headache, neck/eye pain, anticoagulant use, base-line function (which deficits are new?), stool guaiac.

1. **Vascular risk factors:** Smoking, obesity, diabetes, age, angina, MIs, peripheral vascular disease, pregnancy, oral contraceptive use, family history of early MIs or strokes.

2. **Acute exam:** The NIH Stroke Scale is a brief exam useful in acute stroke. Add scores for total. Higher score is worse.

   a. **Level of consciousness:** 0=alert and responsive; 1=arousable to minor stimuli; 2=arousable only to pain; 3=reflex responses or un-arousable.

   b. **Orientation:** Ask pt.'s name and month. Must be exact. 0=both correct; 1=one correct (or dysarthria, intubated, foreign language); 2=neither correct.

   c. **Commands:** Open/close eyes, grip and release non-paretic hand (other one-step command or mimic OK). 0=both correct (OK if impaired by weakness); 1=one correct; 2=neither correct.

   d. **Best gaze:** Horizontal EOM by voluntary or doll's eye test. 0=normal; 1=partial palsy (abnormal in one or both eyes); 2=forced eye deviation or total paresis that cannot be overcome by doll's test).

   e. **Visual field:** Use visual threat if necessary. If monocular, score field of good eye. 0=normal; 1=quadrantanopia, partial hemianopia or extinction; 2=complete hemianopia; 3=blindness.

   f. **Facial palsy:** If stuporous, check grimace to pain. 0=normal; 1=minor paralysis (flat nasolabial fold, asymmetric smile); 2=partial paralysis (lower face); 3=complete paralysis (lower and upper face).

   g. **Motor arms:** Arms outstretched 90 degrees (sitting) or 45 degrees (supine) for 10 sec. Encourage best effort. 0=no drift x 10 sec. 1=drift but doesn't hit bed; 2= some antigravity effort, but can't sustain; 3=no antigravity effort, but even minimal movement counts; 4=no movement at all; X=unable to assess due to amputation, fracture, etc.

   h. **Motor legs:** Score like "Motor arms," above.

   i. **Limb ataxia:** Check finger-nose and heel-shin; score only if out of proportion to paresis. 0=no ataxia (or aphasia, hemiplegic); 1=ataxia in arm or leg; 2=ataxia in arm AND leg; X=unable to assess as above.

   j. **Sensory:** Use pin. Check grimace or withdrawal if stuporous. Score only stroke-related losses. 0=normal; 1=mild-moderate unilateral loss but patient aware of touch (or aphasic or confused); 2=total unilateral loss; pt. unaware of touch; 3=bilateral loss or coma.

   k. **Best language:** Describe picture; name objects; read sentences. May use repeating, writing, stereognosis. 0=normal; 1=mild-moderate aphasia (but comprehensible); 2=severe aphasia (almost no information exchanged); 3=mute, no one-step commands, coma.

   l. **Dysarthria:** Read list of words. 0=normal; 1=mild-moderate slur-ring; 2=severe, unintelligible, or mute; X=intubation or mechanical

barrier.
  m. **Extinction/neglect:** Simultaneously touch patient on both hands, show fingers in both visual fields, ask about deficit, left hand. 0=normal; 1=neglects or extinguishes to double stimulation in any modality; 2=profound neglect in more than one modality.
  3. **Detailed exam:** See sx of specific stroke syndromes, p. 22.
D. **DDx of stroke:** Cerebral bleed, spinal cord lesion, peripheral nerve injury (e.g. Bell's palsy, Saturday night palsy), Todd's paralysis, MS flare, vasculitis, hemiplegic migraine, transient global amnesia, venous infarct, hypoglycemia.
E. **Causes of stroke:**
  1. **Embolus:**
    a. **Cardiac:** About 60% of all strokes. 20% will have known source; 40% cryptogenic. Causes: A fib, valve dz, LV clot (MI, cardiomyopathy), endocarditis, myxoma, hypercoagulable state (see p. 155).
    b. **Paradoxical embolus:** Via patent foramen ovale, atrial or ventricular septal defect; or clot from lung.
    c. **Artery-to-artery embolus:** e.g. from carotid plaque.
    d. **Other:** Fat or air embolus.
  2. **Thrombosis:**
    a. **Large artery:** (About 15% of strokes) Arterial dissection, atherosclerosis.
    b. **Penetrating artery:** (About 25%) Hypertensive lipohyalinosis (lacunar).
    c. **Venous thrombosis:** See p. 98.
  3. **Coagulopathy or platelet disorder.** See p. 155.
  4. **Vasculopathy:** Infectious (syphilis, TB, etc.), drug abuse, collagen vascular dz, moya-moya dz, homocysteinuria, Takayasu's dz, Churg-Strauss dz.
F. **Transient ischemic attack vs. stroke.** TIA was originally defined as a deficit lasting < 24h; now it also usually connotes a normal MRI. Diagnostic workup for TIA is similar to stroke. For acute or recurrent TIAs, strongly consider anticoagulation until workup is complete.
  1. **Embolic TIA:** Sx usually of cortical ischemia, last minutes to hours, before embolus breaks up.
  2. **Low-flow TIA:** Sx usually of watershed ischemia, often blood-pressure dependent.
  3. **Lacunar TIA:** Sx usually of subcortical ischemia, often stuttering or stereotyped.
  4. **Amyloid angiopathy:** Sx of cortical dysfunction, often spreading to adjacent body parts over a few minutes.
G. **Tests:**
  1. **Blood:** Glucose, CBC, PT, PTT (bid on heparin), ESR; consider cholesterol, hypercoagulability panel, anticardiolipin Ab, D-dimer, fibrinogen, RPR, urine homocysteine. Note: CPK rises 4-7 d. post stroke.
  2. **Emergent head CT:** On admission, to rule out bleed.
  3. **Follow-up scan:** To assess stroke territory, e.g. MRI with diffusion-weighted image, or CT in 72 h if no MRI. Consider diffusion-perfusion MRI to look for territory at risk in patient whose exam is

fluctuating, or iron-susceptibility sequence to rule out spells from amyloid angiopathy.

4. **Vascular studies:** Head and neck ultrasound, MRA, or CT angiogram. Consider conventional angiogram.
5. **Cardiac workup:** EKG; consider echocardiogram + bubble study, or TEE, to rule out LV clot, patent foramen ovale. Holter to rule out A fib. Eventually get an ETT because TIA = high risk factor for MI.

H. Rx of stroke

1. **Consider emergent thrombolysis:** Various protocols exist. If available, get an emergent CT angiogram of the vessel in question.
   a. **Contraindications:** Blood or changes on head CT, small or resolving deficit, seizure at symptom onset, signs of SAH, recent bleeding or surgery, abnormal coagulation factors, uncontrollable HTN, very abnormal serum glucose.
   b. **IV tissue plasminogen activator:** Give < 3 h after symptom onset. 0.9 mg/kg up to 90 mg, 10% of total dose as IV bolus, and remainder IV over 60 min.
   c. **Intraarterial streptokinase:** Experimental. Given with angiographic guidance at site of clot, less than 6 h after symptom onset for anterior circulation clot; 12 h for posterior circulation clot.
   d. **Blood pressure management after lysis:** Keep SBP < 180, DBP < 105, with labetalol or nitroprusside if necessary.
2. **Anticoagulants:** For doses, see p. 126.
   a. **Aspirin:** If no bleed on CT, and pt. is not a candidate for thrombolysis, chew 325 mg.
   b. **IV heparin** (if no cerebral bleed): Loading boluses (e.g. 3,000-5,000 unit) <u>only</u> if brainstem ischemia or fluctuating exam.
   c. **Consider long-term anticoagulation:**
      1) **Indications for warfarin:** Atrial fibrillation, mechanical heart valve, carotid or vertebral dissection; possibly prevention of stroke recurrence, embolus of unknown origin, or inoperable severe cerebrovascular stenosis.
      2) **Goal PT INR** = 2-3 for most indications, but 3-4.5 for metal heart valves.
3. **Treat hyperglycemia** > 170 to decrease oxidative metabolism.
4. **Drugs to avoid:** haloperidol, benzodiazepines, α–antagonists.
5. **Orders:**
   a. **SBP** 140-200, or about 20 points higher than pt.'s baseline. Consider keeping pt. flat if there is unstable brainstem ischemia. Try β–blockers first, then α–blockers, then ACE-I.
   b. **Edema:** Consider fluid restriction. If pt. needs IV fluids, give hypertonic D5 NS; aim for hypertonic isovolemia.
   c. **Avoid fever:** e.g. with acetaminophen or cooling blanket.
   d. **Aspiration precautions**.
   e. **bid PTT;** Guaiac stools on heparin.
   f. **Physical and occupational therapy**, but not acutely after stroke, as there is evidence that early PT may extend infarct damage.
6. **Indications for carotid endarterectomy**
   a. **Carotid stenosis:** greater than 70% (debatable between 50 to 70%).

  b. **Deficit:** TIA or infarct in vascular territory distal to lesion.
  c. **No distal stenoses:** Downstream from lesion.
  d. **Good surgical candidate:** No serious cardiac disorders (see p. 173.)
  e. **Stable CNS:** No intracerebral hemorrhage or extensive fresh infarct.

I. **Vascular territories and stroke syndromes**
  1. **See also:** Angiographic anatomy, p. 142.
  2. **Anterior vs. posterior circulation:** The latter are more dangerous. Evidence for posterior ischemia includes bilateral or crossed sensorimotor signs, crossed dissociation of proprioception from pain sensation, cerebellar signs, stupor or coma, lower cranial nerve deficits.
  3. **Middle cerebral artery:**
    a. **Superior division:** Arm or face weakness > leg, Broca's aphasia.
    b. **Inferior division:** Mild or transient motor/sensory deficit, Wernicke's aphasia, neglect, sometimes field cut (Meyer's loop infarct causes superior quadrantanopsia, not hemianopsia), Gerstmann's syndrome: (dominant inferior parietal lobule, with acalculia, L-R dissociation, finger agnosia, agraphia).
  4. **Anterior cerebral artery:** Contralateral leg weak, grasp reflex, Gegenhalten, abulia, gait disorder, perseveration, urinary incontinence. Sometimes bilateral if both ACAs have common origin.
  5. **ACA-MCA watershed:** Contralateral trunk > limb weakness.
  6. **MCA-PCA watershed:** Parietal lobe dysfunction.
  7. **Posterior cerebral artery:** Contralateral field cut. Sometimes memory loss, color anomia, alexia without agraphia, hemisensory loss, mild hemiparesis. Spatial disorientation is nondominant superior parietal lobule.
    a. **Watch for brainstem ischemia:** PCA stroke can be the beginning of a top-of-the-basilar syndrome.
    b. **Uncal herniation** can pinch off PCAs.
  8. **Subcortical arteries:**
    a. **Medial striates:** Include recurrent artery of Heubner. See Broca's aphasia, mild hemiparesis arm > leg, proximal > distal. Comes off ACA or A-comm to anterior hypothalamus, globus pallidus, putamen, caudate nucleus.
    b. **Anterior choroidal and other lenticulostriates:** Contralateral sensorimotor loss, homonymous hemianopsia. The anterior choroidal comes off ICA to posterior limb of internal capsule, cerebral peduncle, and medial globus pallidus.
  9. **Basilar artery:** Infarct causes pontine and cerebellar signs.
    a. **Occlusion:** Frequently bilateral signs, e.g. quadriplegia, conjugate horizontal gaze palsies, coma, "locked-in" syndrome.
    b. **"Top of the basilar" embolus:** Classically see oculomotor palsy, dorsal midbrain syndrome, bilateral thalamic stroke. Emboli from basilar clot can cause occipital infarcts with field cuts, thalamic infarcts with poor arousal or memory loss, cerebellar infarcts with ipsilateral ataxia, brainstem infarcts with contralateral hemiplegia but ipsilateral horizontal gaze palsy (opposite of cerebral lesion), internuclear ophthalmoplegia, palatal myoclonus, etc.

10. **Midbrain strokes:** From occlusion of basilar branches. Damage to oculomotor, Edinger-Westphal, red, trochlear, or lateral geniculate nuclei; reticular activating system.
    a. **Dorsal midbrain syndrome:** Supranuclear upgaze paralysis, light-near dissociation, convergence paralysis.
    b. **Rostral interstitial nucleus:** Blood = from branch of PCA. Infarct of single side can give bilateral upgaze palsy because also infarct crossing fibers en passant.
    c. **Ventral midbrain syndrome:** Bilateral downgaze paralysis, paralysis of convergence, obtundation.
11. **Pontine strokes:** From occlusion of basilar branches. Damage to motor and sensory nuclei of nerves V, VII and VIII, reticular activating system.
    a. **"Locked-in" syndrome:** From basis pontis lesion, sparing tegmentum.
12. **Cerebellar strokes:** Vertigo, N/V, nystagmus, ataxia, poor smooth pursuit, often headache; often with brainstem signs including ipsilateral hearing loss, ipsilateral Horner's syndrome, contralateral pain and temperature loss. <u>Large cerebellar strokes are an emergency</u>, because of the risk of herniation. Consider neurosurgical decompression. Pt. can die within hours of first brainstem signs. SCA and AICA are off basilar; PICA off vertebral.
    a. **Superior cerebellar artery:** Ataxia. Usually embolic. Rarely causes hydrocephalus (7%).
    b. **Posterior inferior cerebellar artery:** Vertigo, N/V. Often with lateral medullary syndrome (see below). 50% embolic, 50% from vertebral stenosis. If whole territory is infarcted, there's a 25% risk of hydrocephalus.
    c. **Anterior inferior cerebellar artery:** Rare; usually from thrombosis; usually with brainstem infarct too. Hearing loss, weak/numb face, ataxia, vertigo.
13. **Medullary stroke:** From vertebral artery lesion. Signs of damage to nerves VIII, IX-XII, spinal tract, and nucleus of V. Hemiparesis implies more medial involvement, or higher lesion.
    a. **Lateral medullary syndrome** (Wallenberg's):
        1) **Vestibular signs:** Vertigo, N/V, nystagmus, diplopia.
        2) **Sensory signs:** Sensory loss on <u>ipsilateral</u> face; poor pain and temperature sensation on <u>contralateral</u> body.
        3) **Horner's syndrome:** Ipsilaterally
        4) **Cranial nerves IX, X:** Dysphagia, hoarseness, hiccups, poor gag ipsilaterally.
        5) **Ataxia:** Ipsilateral.
    b. **Medial medullary syndrome:** Ipsilateral tongue weakness and deviation, contralateral hemiparesis, and poor proprioception, but cutaneous sensation spared.
14. **Lacunar syndromes:** Thought to be from hypertensive lipohyalinosis; probably not helped by heparin.
    a. **Typical locations:** In order of decreasing frequency: putamen, caudate, thalamus, pons, internal capsule, corona radiata.
    b. **Pure sensory:** Ventral posterolateral or posteromedial nucleus of

the thalamus.
- c. **Pure motor:** Posterior limb of internal capsule, basis pontis, or cerebral peduncle.
- d. **Ataxic hemiparesis:** Ataxia >>> weakness on same side. Often leg > arm > face. From basis pontis (upper third, midline), or ventral anterior thalamus + adjacent internal capsule, or superior cerebellar peduncle.
- e. **Dysarthria-clumsy hand:** Weak face, dysphagia, and ipsilateral clumsy hand. From lesion of basis pontis, genu of internal capsule, or immediately subcortical white matter.

COMA AND BRAIN DEATH

A. **See also** Trauma, p. 89.
B. **Levels of decreased consciousness:**
  1. **Confusion:** Decreased attention but relatively normal alertness.
  2. **Drowsiness** (~lethargy, somnolence): Arouses to voice and can respond verbally.
  3. **Stupor** (~obtundation): No response to voice, no spontaneous speech. Incomplete but purposive response to pain.
  4. **Coma:** Nonpurposive or no response to pain.
C. **Other alterations in consciousness:** See p. 33.
D. **Initial coma evaluation:** (1) Do cardiopulmonary resuscitation, (2) get IV access, (3) draw blood (include tox screen, ?carbon monoxide level), (4) give dextrose, thiamine, and naloxone, (5) do coma exam (see below), (6) treat suspected high ICP, meningitis, or seizures, (7) do CT scan, (8) treat metabolic problems.
E. **Coma exam:** VS (and note pattern of breathing), cardiac rhythm, response to voice, lids (spontaneously closed?), pupils, eye movements, (spontaneous, doll's, calorics), corneals, grimace to nasal tickle, gag, motor response to pain, tone (lift and drop arm), reflexes.
  1. **Decorticate posturing:**
    a. **Arm:** Flexed elbow, wrist, fingers.
    b. **Leg:** extended and internally rotated leg, with plantar flexion.
  2. **Decerebrate posturing:** (Hypoxia, hypoglycemia can cause)
    a. **Head:** Clenched jaw, extended neck.
    b. **Arm:** Adducted shoulder, extended elbow, pronated wrist, flexed fingers.
    c. **Leg:** Extended and internally rotated leg, plantar flexion.
F. **Glasgow coma scale:** Range 3-15. Add points in each category. Pt. gets 3 points for just being in the room.

Points	Eye opening	Verbal	Motor
6			Obeys
5		Oriented	Localizes pain
4	Spontaneous	Confused	Withdraws to pain
3	To speech	Inappropriate	Flexion (decort.)
2	To pain	Unintelligible	Extensor (decereb.)
1	None	None	None

Table 4. Glasgow Coma Scale.

G. Causes of coma with normal head CT:
   1. **Drug overdose or reaction:** Especially sedatives, anticholinergics, and poisons, but also including neuroleptic malignant syndrome.
   2. **Anoxia or ischemia:** Cardiac arrest, brainstem stroke, fat or cholesterol emboli, DIC, thrombotic thrombocytopenic purpura, vasculitis.
   3. **Trauma:** Diffuse axonal injury, bilateral isodense SDH.
   4. **Metabolic encephalopathy:** Low or high glucose, low or high Na, high Ca, alkalosis, hypercapnia, adrenal crisis, low or high thyroid, uremia, high ammonia, Wernicke's syndrome, hypothermia.
   5. **Infection:** Meningitis, encephalitis, or sepsis.
   6. **Nonconvulsive status epilepticus.**
   7. **Central pontine myelinolysis.**
H. Prognosis in <u>non</u>traumatic coma:
   1. **Confounding factors:** All drug effects, reversible metabolic factors, and hypothermia must be corrected first.
   2. **Prognosis by etiology:** Those with hepatic cause do best, hypoxic-ischemic intermediate, vascular worst.
   3. **Prognosis by neurological exam:**
      a. **Day of presentation:** Look for corneal, pupillary, and oculocephalic (doll's or calorics) responses.
         1) **Absence of 1 of the 3:** 95% of pts. will be vegetative or severely disabled.
         2) **Absence of 2 of the 3:** 99% of pts. will be vegetative or severely disabled.
      b. **Day 1:**
         1) **Spontaneous eye movements:** 99% of pts. who don't have spontaneous conjugate roving eye movements or better will be vegetative or severely disabled.
         2) **Motor withdrawal:** Of pts. with spontaneous eye movements but no purposive withdrawal to pain, 90% will be vegetative or severely disabled.
      c. **Day 3:**
         1) **Motor withdrawal:** Of pts. with no purposive withdrawal to pain, 100% will be vegetative or severely disabled.
         2) **Spontaneous eye opening:** Of pts. who withdraw but keep eyes closed, 80% will be vegetative or severely disabled.
      d. **Day 7:**
         1) **Spontaneous eye opening:** Of pts. who withdraw but keep eyes closed, 100% will be vegetative.
         2) **Obeying commands:** Of pts. with spontaneous eye opening who don't follow commands, about 80% will be vegetative or severely disabled.
      e. **Day 14:**
         1) **Abnormal oculocephalic reflex:**
            a) **Not following commands or opening eyes spontaneously:** 100% vegetative.
            b) **Following commands or opening eyes spontaneously:** 80% vegetative or severely disabled.
         2) **Normal oculocephalic reflex:** Only 20% will be severely disabled or worse.

I. Vegetative state: Similar to coma, but patient may have sleep-wake cycles and eye opening to auditory stimuli, with no awareness of environment or self, no ability to communicate, and no purposive motor activity.

J. Brain death: An attending must see the pt. before declaring brain-dead. If there may be litigation about the death, get legal counsel first. The following criteria should be met:

1. **Known cause**
2. **No hypothermia (< 32°C) or CNS depressants.**
3. **No evidence of brainstem function.**
   a. **Reflexes:** No pupillary, corneal, oculovestibular, gag, or other brainstem reflexes.
   b. **No motor response to deep central pain.** There should be neither decerebrate nor decorticate posturing, but spinal reflexes including flexor withdrawal can be seen after brain death. There should be no change in heart rate to pain.
4. **Apnea test:** Criterion is no spontaneous breaths and $pCO_2 > 60$ (unreliable in pt. with COPD and CO_2 retention).
   a. **Pre-oxygenate:** 15 min of ventilation with 100% O_2 beforehand.
   b. **Disconnect ventilator;** Give O_2 8-12 L/min by tracheal cannula; observe for spontaneous breaths.
   c. **Draw ABG** after about 10 min (depends on pt. stability).
   d. **Terminate test if** $pCO_2 > 60$ (usually takes 6-12 min), pt. breathes, has significant hypotension, cardiac arrhythmia, or O_2 saturation drops below 80%.
5. **Observation period:** Use clinical judgment. Recommendations:
   a. **24 hrs:** For anoxic brain injury and no confirmatory tests.
   b. **12 hrs:** For clear irreversible condition, no confirmatory tests.
   c. **6 hrs:** For clear irreversible condition, confirmatory tests.
6. **Confirmatory tests:** (not necessary)
   a. **Flat EEG:** Isoelectric at high gain.
   b. **Absent cerebral blood flow:** e.g. by transcranial ultrasound, or an ICP > SBP for 1 h.

K. Organ and tissue donation:

1. **Eligibility criteria:** Candidates may be any age. There are additional exclusion criteria not listed below (e.g. HIV infection), but call the transplant coordinator and let him or her decide.
   a. **Organ donation:** Brain dead, intact circulation, ventilated.
   b. **Tissue donation:** Anyone with irreversible absence of respiration and circulation.
2. **Transplant coordinator:** Call early: 1-800-446-6362, even if you haven't yet asked the family—the organ bank won't approach the family without your permission.
3. **When and how to ask the family:** In some states, you ask all families of eligible donors about organ donation. Especially in the ICU, the nurses have had much experience with this. Ask their advice, if possible.
4. **Management after brain death for organ donation:** The transplant team will help once the pt. is declared braindead. Before that, of course, you should treat the pt. with his or her best interest in mind only.

CRANIAL NERVES

A. See also: BRAINSTEM ANATOMY, p. 15.

	CNS nucleus	**Function**
I	Olfactory bulb	Smell
II	Retina; lateral geniculate nu	Vision, p. 37
III	Oculomotor nu. (somatic motor)	EOM except sup. oblique and lat. rectus, p. 39
	Edinger-Westphal (PSNS)	Pupillary constriction, p. 36
IV	Trochlear nu.	Superior oblique muscle, p. 39
V	Spinal and main sensory nu.	Sensory from face, dura, tympani
	Mesencephalic nu.	Mechanoreceptors of face, mouth
	Trigeminal motor nu.	Muscles of chewing, tensor tymp.
VI	Abducens nu.	Lateral rectus muscle, p. 39
VII	Facial motor nu.	Facial expression and stapedius
	Spinal trigeminal nu.	Ear and tympanic memb. sensation
	Solitary nu.	Taste from ant. 2/3 of tongue
	Sup. salivatory nu.	Salivation and lacrimation
VIII	Cochlear nu.	Hearing (p. 45)
	Vestibular nu.	Balance (p. 98)
IX	Nu. ambiguus	Pharyngeal muscles
	Spinal trigeminal nu.	Sensation of ear, post. 1/3 of tongue
	Solitary nu.	Taste from post. 1/3 tongue
	Solitary and spinal trigem.	Carotid, oropharynx sensation
	Inf. salivatory nu.	Parotid gland secretion
X	Nu. ambiguus	Larynx/pharynx muscles
	Spinal trigeminal nu.	Sensory from external ear
	Solitary nu.	Taste buds of epiglottis
	Solitary and spinal trigeminal nu.	Larynx/pharynx sensation; PSNS from chest and abdomen
	Dorsal motor nu.	PSNS to chest and abdomen
XI	Nu ambiguus	Larynx and pharynx muscles
	Accessory nu.	Sternocleidomastoid and trapezius
XII	Hypoglossal nu.	Intrinsic tongue muscles

Table 5. Cranial nerve nuclei and their functions.

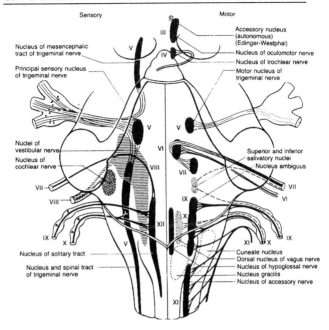

Figure 5. Cranial nerve nuclei. (From Duus P. *Topical Diagnosis in Neurology.* New York: Thieme, 1983:105, with permission.).

DEMYELINATING DISEASE

A. Multiple sclerosis: Pt. should have two attacks lasting > 24 h, in two different locations, separated by more than a month. Disease is classified as definite or probable. Course may be relapsing or progressive.

  1. H&P:

  a. **Common presenting sx:** Optic neuritis, weakness and numbness, diplopia, vertigo, myelitis, urinary retention. Sx worse with heat.

  b. **Other MS sx:** Urinary retention, pain, fatigue, Lhermitte's phenomenon (tingling on neck flexion), internuclear ophthalmoplegia, cognitive changes. Weakness frequently worst in hands and hips.

  c. **MS flare:** Usually subacute (> 1 wk) deterioration. Acute (1-3 d) deterioration suggests an infection that is briefly exacerbating MS sx—does the pt. use catheters?

  2. DDx:

  a. **DDx of MS:** Acute disseminated encephalomyelitis, cervical cord compression, CNS lymphomas and gliomas, vasculitis, lupus, myelitis, infection (HIV, Lyme), neurosarcoid, Chiari malformations, B_{12} deficiency, arylsulfatase or hexosaminidase A deficiencies, mitochondrial dzs,....

    b. DDx of MS attack in pt. with known MS: Infection (<u>bladder</u> > teeth > URI); cervical or lumbar disc herniation, entrapment neuropathy,....

3. Tests:

    a. Initial workup:

        1) **MRI + contrast:** See p. 151. Pts. with a first MS-like neurological event and significant white-matter lesions on MRI have a 5-year incidence of MS about 80%. If no lesions, risk is about 5%.

        2) **Consider:** CSF IgG and oligoclonal bands, Lyme titer, B_{12} level, HIV test, ESR, ANA, ACE level.

    b. MS attack: CBC, urinalysis, and ESR to help r/o infection that could mimic an attack; consider tests to r/o disc herniation or entrapment neuropathy.

4. Rx of MS attack: Don't treat mild sensory attacks.

    a. High-dose steroids: e.g. methylprednisolone IV in D5 W over 4-6 h qd: 1000 mg in 1000 ml x 5 d ± prednisone taper.

    b. Prevention of steroid side effects: See p. 138.

5. To slow MS progression:

    a. β-interferon: Approved for relapsing-remitting MS. Avonex (β-IFN 1a, given 6 million U IM qwk) may be better tolerated than Betaseron (β-IFN 1b).

    b. Glatiramer (Copaxone): Fragments of myelin basic protein. 20 mg SC qd.

    c. Cyclophosphamide (Cytoxan): Controversial. For aggressively progressive MS.

    d. Other immunosuppressants.

6. Symptomatic therapy: See rx for spasticity, p. 139; pain, p. 124; tremor, p. 62; and spastic bladder or bladder-sphincter dyssynergia, p. 96. Fatigue may respond to amantidine 100 mg PO bid. Brief, painful, focal seizures sometimes resolve after a few weeks of low-dose anticonvulsant.

B. Other central demyelinating conditions:

1. Acute disseminated encephalomyelitis (ADEM): Multifocal demyelination similar to MS but acute, monophasic, sometimes postinfectious.

    a. H&P: Recent viral infection or vaccination.

    b. DDx: Infectious encephalomyelitis.

    c. Rx: Consider steroids, plasmapheresis.

2. Acute hemorrhagic leukoencephalitis: A hyperacute ADEM, often with fever, seizures, obtundation.

3. Transverse myelitis: Isolated spinal cord dysfunction without compressive lesion, often following febrile illness.

4. Cerebellitis: See p. 114.

5. Brainstem (Bickerstaff's) encephalitis : Adolescents and young adults.

C. Guillain-Barré syndrome

1. <u>GBS is an emergency</u>: Because of the danger of sudden respiratory collapse, even in pts. without severe limb weakness.

2. AKA: Acute idiopathic demyelinating polyradiculoneuritis (AIDP, as opposed to CIDP, below.)

3. H&P: Virus, vaccination, or surgery in previous 1-3 wk; pregnancy. Rapid symmetric weakness, weak DTRs, facial diplegia, poor swallowing or breathing, stocking/glove numbness hands and feet. Sometimes proximal > distal (vs. other peripheral neuropathies), ANS instability; diffuse back pain.

4. Variants:
  a. Miller Fisher variant: Areflexia, sensory ataxia, ophthalmoparesis.
  b. Polyneuritis cranialis: A variant that often presents with bifacial weakness.
  c. Acute pan-dysautonomia: ANS instability, papilledema, upgoing toes. No meningeal signs.

5. Tests:
  a. Respiratory: Vital capacity tid. Remember that O_2 saturation is not sensitive; pt. will become hypercarbic before becoming hypoxic.
  b. Blood: β-HCG, heterophile Ab and EBV titers, *Campylobacter*, HIV, CMV, RF, ANA, hepatitis titers.
  c. NCS: Conduction block, usually low velocity, high latency, decreased F-wave conduction. Poor correlation with sx; can be nl early in dz).
  d. Biopsy shows focal demyelination. Consider biopsy only if dx unclear.
  e. CSF: Protein usually up after 1st few days. Cell count usually normal; sometimes 10-100 monocytes.

6. DDx of GBS: CIDP, other neuropathies (see p. 72); neuromuscular problem, e.g. myasthenia or botulism, Lyme, MS, foramen magnum or other spine tumor, polio, hypophosphatemia (during long course of parenteral nutrition), tick paralysis,....

7. Rx: Intubate if vital capacity < 15 ml/kg or 0.6 L, or higher if falling fast. Plasmapheresis (ANS instability is a relative contraindication) or IV Ig. No role for steroids (though helps CIDP). Protect eyes from drying. Back pain may require narcotics. Watch for SIADH.
  a. Prognosis: 35% have permanent deficit, 10% have relapse, 50% nadir in 1 wk, 90% in 1 mo. Axonal variants do worse. Amplitude < 250 do worse (implies more distal conduction block).

D. Chronic inflammatory demyelinating polyradiculoneuropathy (CIDP):
  1. H&P: Peak incidence age 50-60; progressive or relapsing weakness > 2 mo., usually legs > arms, depressed DTRs, stocking-glove numbness or tingling.
  2. DDx: Systemic dz, toxin exposure, familial neuropathy.
  3. Tests: NCS show demyelination, CSF protein > 45 mg/dl, cell count < $10/\mu l$, sural nerve biopsy shows de- and re-myelination with perivascular inflammation.
  4. Rx: Steroids, plasma exchange, IV Ig.

DYSARTHRIA AND DYSPHAGIA

A. **Dysarthria:** Abnormal articulation, as opposed to aphasia.
  1. **H&P:** Abnormal articulation, rhythm, or volume. Ask about diurnal fluctuations (suggests myasthenia), improvement with alcohol (suggests essential tremor). Assess palatal elevation when pt. says a long "a" or "coca-cola." Assess ability to hold a tone or sing. Look especially for other cranial nerve signs, dysmetria, tremor, dystonia, or spasticity.
  2. **Related conditions:**
     a. **Spasmodic dysphonia:** Often associated with dystonia. Adductor dysphonia is choppy and strained; adductor dysphonia is breathy, interspersed with whispering. Botulinum toxin can help.
     b. **Dysfluency:** Includes stuttering, cluttering, palilalia.
  3. **Tests:** MRI; consider EMG of orofacial muscles (painful).
  4. **DDx:** Maxillofacial lesion, aphasia, intoxication, or delirium.
  5. **Causes:** See also bulbar vs. pseudobulbar palsy, p. 100.
     a. **Peripheral** (flaccid): Myasthenia, polyneuritis, myopathy, cranial nerve lesions.
     b. **Central:** Spastic (corticospinal tract damage), ataxic (cerebellar lesion), bradykinetic (parkinsonism), hyperkinetic (chorea, dystonia).
     c. **Mixed:** Spastic-flaccid (ALS), spastic-ataxic (MS, Wilson's dz, encephalitis).
  6. **Rx:** Treat underlying dz.
B. **Dysphagia:** Abnormal swallowing.
  1. **H&P:** Choking, coughing after swallowing, weight loss, recurrent pneumonias. Is it worse with liquids or solids? Watch pt. swallow water, assess gag, other cranial nerves, motor exam.
  2. **Tests:** "Swallowing study" (cine-esophogram). Brain scan. CXR if you suspect aspiration pneumonia.
  3. **Causes:**
     a. **Nonneurological:** Esophageal mass, scleroderma, achalasia, esophageal spasm, Sjögren's syndrome.
     b. **Neurological:** Upper or lower motor neuron lesion (stroke, brainstem mass, etc.), ALS, neuropathy, MS, myasthenia, Chiari malformation, syringobulbia, myopathy, Parkinson's dz, spinocerebellar degeneration, tardive dyskinesia, cerebral palsy.
  4. **Rx:** "Aspiration precautions," swallowing therapy, dysphagia diets (e.g. purees), thickened liquids, nasogastric or gastric tube.

ELECTROENCEPHALOGRAPHY

A. **Indications:** Confirming, localizing, or classifying seizures. Aiding in the diagnosis of Creutzfeldt-Jacob dz and encephalitis. A normal EEG never rules out the possibility of seizures.
B. **Montages:**
  1. **Bipolar:** Good for localization, but it distorts widely distributed potentials, e.g. vertex waves. Location of spike = at phase reversal.
  2. **Referential:** Good for sleep studies. More EKG artifact. Location of

spike = at max amplitude.

C. Studies:
   1. **Routine.**
   2. **Sleep-deprived:** More sensitive for epileptiform activity, which is seen especially in sleep-wake transitions.
   3. **Continuous:** Indications include anticonvulsant coma in status epilepticus, nonconvulsive status, capturing seizures to determine the hemisphere in which the seizure began (for epilepsy surgery), and distinguishing seizures from pseudoseizures.

D. Normal rhythms:
   1. **Alpha:** 8-12 Hz, posterior. Resting rhythm of thalamus. Disappears when eyes open, or when drowsy.
   2. **Beta:** Fast 20-40 Hz, anterior. Cortical activity during alertness.
   3. **Theta:** 4-8 Hz. Normal during drowsiness/sleep; abnormal when alert.
   4. **Delta:** < 4 Hz. Normal during drowsiness/sleep; abnormal when alert.
   5. **Sleep:** Generalized slowing, vertex waves, K complexes, sleep spindles (14 Hz), drowsy hypersynchrony.
   6. **Normal effects of stimulation:**
      a. **Hyperventilation:** Can cause generalized slowing in normals.
      b. **Photic stimulation:** Occipital driving; often more with eyes closed.

E. Abnormal rhythms:
   1. **Slowing:** Theta or delta while alert. Nonspecific if generalized; may help localize lesion if focal.
   2. **Seizure:** High-voltage, chaotic or rhythmic, focal or generalized.
   3. **Spikes and sharp waves:** Interictal evidence for epilepsy.
   4. **Frontal intermittent rhythmic delta activity:** Nonspecific encephalopathy.
   5. **Diffuse periodic sharps:** DDx = Creutzfeldt-Jacob dz, lithium toxicity, baclofen toxicity, metabolic encephalopathy, subacute sclerosing panencephalitis (has complexes with longer periodicity).
   6. **Periodic lateralized epileptiform discharges:** Don't try to eradicate them; just aim for normal anticonvulsant levels.
   7. **Triphasic waves:** Usually from metabolic abnormality, although they look ictal.

ELECTROMYOGRAPHY AND NERVE CONDUCTION STUDIES

	Conduction Velocity (%)	Amplitude	F-, H latency	Distal latency	Fibrillations
Axonal neuropathy	>70	↓	~↑	nl	↑
Demyel. neuropathy	<50	~↓	↑	~↑	Variable
Lower motor neuron dz	>70	↓ Motor	~↑	nl	↑
Upper motor neuron dz	nl	nl	nl	nl	None
Radiculopathy	>80	~↓	↑	nl	↑
Neuromusc. jcn. defect	nl	nl/↓	nl	nl	None
Myopathy	nl	~↓	nl	nl	None

Table 6. EMG findings in neuromuscular diseases.

A. Ordering tests: Always give tentative dx; specify muscles, nerves of in-

terest.
- B. **Nerve conduction studies:** Record amplitude, duration, shape, and latency of waveform.
  - 1. **Motor NCS:** Stimulate motor nerve, record muscle compound muscle action potential (CMAP).
    - a. **F-wave:** Small peak after first (M) wave, caused by antidromic stimulation of motor neuron. F-wave delayed in proximal neuropathies, e.g. DM, GBS; also in motor neuron dz and radiculopathy.
    - b. **H-reflex:** CMAP from stimulation of sensory nerve, via monosynaptic reflex arc. Always tested in tibia: dorsal and ventral S1 roots. H-reflex delayed and small if proximal sensory or motor axon damage.
    - c. **Repetitive stimulation:**
      - 1) **Myasthenia:**. Repetitive 3-Hz stimulation of proximal muscle at rest makes CMAP get smaller. With exercise, CMAP size recovers in a few seconds, but then worsens in 2-4 min
      - 2) **Lambert-Eaton syndrome:**, Baseline CMAP small, and gets smaller with repetitive 3-Hz stimulation. With exercise, CMAP size greatly increases in a few sec, but then worsens in 2-4 min.
      - 3) **Botulism:** Baseline CMAP very small; gets smaller with repetitive 3-Hz stimulation; no change with exercise.
  - 2. **Sensory NCS:** Stimulate a nerve and record its sensory nerve action potential (SNAP) and another point along the nerve.
- C. **Electromyography:** (also called needle study)
  - 1. **Insertional activity:** Triggered by needle movement. It is decreased in denervation, myotonia, some myopathies (especially inflammatory myopathies), periodic paralysis during the paralysis, and muscle fibrosis.
  - 2. **Spontaneous activity:** Many possible abnormal findings, including fibrillation potentials, fasciculation potentials, myotonic discharges, decreased or increased recruitment, etc.

ENCEPHALOPATHY, DELIRIUM, AND DEMENTIA

- A. **See also:** Metabolic, toxic, and deficiency disorders, p. 55.
- B. **Management of agitation**
  - 1. **Orders:** Posey vest or soft restraints qhs, aspiration precautions, consult social services for long-term placement if necessary.
  - 2. **Drugs:** If neurological exam nonfocal, consider lorazepam or haloperidol.
  - 3. **Emergent chemical restraint:** Haloperidol 5 mg IM, lorazepam 2 mg IM, diphenhydramine 50 mg IM. Avoid haloperidol in patients with extrapyramidal dz.
  - 4. **Chronic agitation:** Consider haloperidol 0.5 mg qhs or bid, or an atypical neuroleptic such as risperidone.
- C. **Delirium:** Agitated confusion, usually with the implication of acute metabolic cause. Usually slurred speech, often frank hallucinations, motor signs (tremor, myoclonus, asterixis), sometimes seizures.
  - 1. **DDx:** Hypoxia, hypercapnia, electrolytes, glucose, drug overdose or withdrawal, sepsis, meningitis, encephalitis, high ammonia, uremia,

Wernicke's syndrome. Consider also depression, psychosis, thyroid storm, transient global amnesia, nonconvulsive status epilepticus, posterior leukoencephalopathy,....

2. **Tests:** Consider head CT, ABG, EKG, electrolytes, BUN, Cr, Ca, ammonia, toxin screen, CBC, ESR, LP, EEG.

D. **Encephalopathy:** Nonspecific term for diffuse brain dysfunction, often from systemic process, that is not a classic dementia.

1. **Reversible causes of subacute or chronic encephalopathy:** Pseudo-dementia of depression, metabolic delirium, bilateral SDH, normal pressure hydrocephalus, vasculitis, lymphoma, metabolic, tumor (especially falx meningioma), thyroid, B_{12}, thiamine, infection (especially HIV, syphilis, fungal).

2. **Creutzfeldt-Jacob dz:** Sporadic or familial buildup of prion protein particles.

   a. **H&P:** Variable combinations of myoclonus, dementia, and ataxia, progresses to death in 6 mo-2 yr.

   b. **Tests:** Brain biopsy shows spongiform encephalopathy. EEG shows diffuse periodic sharps. MRI may show basal ganglia and white matter lesions. Experimental assays for 14-3-3 protein in CSF are available (also high in encephalitis and some gliomas).

   c. **Precautions:** Transmissible only when infected neural tissue contacts an open wound. However, the agent is not inactivated by standard sterilization techniques.

E. **Dementia:** Chronic selective loss of higher cortical functions, especially memory and naming. Pt. may be disoriented acutely at night, but frank hallucinations rare.

1. **H&P:** Education, baseline personality, activities of daily living, falls, incontinence, drug changes, h/o depression. Check primitive reflexes. See also Mini-Mental Status Exam, p. 77.

2. **Tests:** Head CT, SMA20, CBC, VDRL, ESR, TSH, B_{12}. Consider HIV test, LP, EEG, heavy metal screen, brain biopsy

3. **Potentially reversible causes:** See Encephalopathy, above.

4. **Normal pressure hydrocephalus:**

   a. **H&P:** Frontal gait (see p. 59), incontinence (from abulia or not being able to get to bathroom), dementia (frontal, abulic, vs. Alzheimer's type). No headache or papilledema.

   b. **Tests:** Serial LPs (not perfectly sensitive, pt. can need up to 3 mo of VP shunt before improving). Consider ICP monitor x 48 h to look for plateau waves (V or A). Consider trial of Sinemet to rule out Parkinson's dz.

   c. **Rx of NPH:** Ventriculoperitoneal shunt. Risk is SDH (vessels already stretched by atrophy). Gait apraxia responds best; dementia worst, especially if long-standing.

5. **Irreversible causes:**

   a. **Cortical:**

      1) **Alzheimer's dz (AD):** Usually with triad of aphasia, apraxia, and agnosia.

      2) **Lewy body dz:** More episodic delirium, psychiatric features (hallucinations, depression), and extrapyramidal features than AD. May benefit from low-dose Sinemet or a dopamine agonist

in combination with an atypical neuroleptic e.g. quetiapine. Avoid typical neuroleptics.

   3) **Pick's dz:** More personality change, less aphasia or amnesia than AD.
   4) **Multiple sclerosis:** Often mild, with frontal disinhibition.
   b. **Subcortical:** Slowed responses, often with motor problems. Binswanger's dz (periventricular demyelination), Huntington's dz, HIV dementia complex, progressive supranuclear palsy, Parkinson's dz.
   c. **Mixed:** Multi-infarct dementia, Creutzfeldt-Jacob dz.
   d. **Rx:** Social services, antidepressants (avoid TCAs), neuroleptics such as haloperidol, thioridazine, or short-acting benzodiazepines for aggression. Donepizil (Aricept) may slightly slow cognitive decline.

EVOKED POTENTIALS

A. **General:** AKA evoked responses. Record latency, amplitude, R/L discrepancies from scalp during stimulation of sensory modalities.
   1. **Indications:** To detect clinically silent lesions, objective proof of sensory deficits.
B. **Visual evoked responses (VERs):** Stimulus is checkerboard pattern. P100 is prolonged in retinal or optic nerve lesion; need electroretinograms (ERGs) to differentiate between the two.
C. **Somatosensory Evoked Potentials (SSEPs):** Stimulate median or posterior tibial nerve. Prolonged if lesion of nerve, spinal cord, brainstem, ~ cortex.
D. **Brainstem auditory evoked responses (BSAERs):** 7 waves; only I, III, and V are important. I is from cranial nerve VIII, III = bilateral superior olive, V = inferior colliculus, IPL = interpeak latency.
   1. **All waves absent:** Suggests peripheral deafness.
   2. **I-III prolonged** (or III absent): Suggests pontomedullary junction lesion, e.g. MS, cerebellopontine angle tumor, pontine glioma, brainstem infarct.
   3. **III-V prolonged** (or V absent): Pons/midbrain lesion, e.g. MS, extrinsic mass compressing brainstem (includes contralateral CPA tumor).
   4. **All waves prolonged:** Suggests diffuse dz, e.g. MS, big glioma. Not usually metabolic.

EYES AND VISION

A. **Lids**
   1. **Ptosis** (lid droop):
      a. **Unilateral ptosis:** Horner's syndrome, 3rd nerve palsy, myasthenia (varies with fatigue), trauma. Lower lid sag from 7th nerve palsy can mask ptosis.
      b. **Bilateral ptosis:** Nuclear 3rd nerve lesion, myasthenia, progressive external ophthalmoplegia, age-related periorbital atrophy, redundant lid tissue, oculopharyngeal dystrophy, bilateral third palsy.

    2. Blink rate: Decreased in extrapyramidal bradykinetic syndromes. These pts. often cannot suppress blinks to repeated forehead tap (Myerson's sign), and may have blepharoclonus (lid fluttering) with eyes closed.

    3. Lid retraction: Consider dorsal midbrain syndrome; hyperthyroidism (often with lid lag as pt. looks down), chronic steroids.

B. Exophthalmos

    1. AKA: Proptosis.

    2. DDx: Carotid cavernous fistula (usually pulsatile), tumor, hyperthyroidism, infection, inflammation, hemorrhage, 3rd nerve palsy (via rectus relaxation), carotid sinus occlusion.

C. Horner's syndrome:

    1. H&P:

        a. Ptosis: An ID photo can show if it's old.

        b. Miosis (small pupil): Worse in dark (vs. 3rd nerve lesion -- worse in light). There should be a dilation lag when lights are turned off.

        c. Anhidrosis: Seen if lesion is in nerve before the sweat afferents leave with ext. carotid artery. Wipe on iodine bilaterally and let it dry; then put starch from a glove on top. Sweat will turn it purple.

    2. Tests for localization:

        a. Cocaine test: Confirms Horner's syndrome: dilates normal pupil only. Blocks reuptake so no effect unless norepinephrine being released at pupil.

        b. Hydroxyamphetamine test: Dilates Horner's syndrome pupils only if 3rd order neurons are intact, because it is an indirect agonist.

    3. Causes of isolated Horner's syndrome:

        a. Third-order lesion: Usually idiopathic (if congenital, iris is often heterochromic).

        b. First and 2nd-order: Malignancy (including Pancoast) > cluster HA > vascular (dissection, cavernous thrombosis, ischemia) > cervical disk > trauma (including thoracic surgery) > meningitis > PTX > intrinsic brainstem lesion (usually with other findings).

D. Fundi

    1. Papilledema: Look for venous pulsations, acuity, fields, tenderness to eye pressure.

        a. DDx bilateral papilledema: High ICP, pseudotumor cerebri, metabolic problems,...

        b. DDx unilateral papilledema:

            1) **Visual loss and pain:** Neuritis, infection, other inflammation.

            2) **Visual loss, no pain:** Ant. ischemic optic neuropathy, e.g. from diabetes, embolus, polycythemia.

            3) **With no visual loss:** High ICP with contralateral optic atrophy e.g. from compression (Foster-Kennedy syndrome).

    2. Optic atrophy: Glaucoma, past neuritis; chronic papilledema.

E. Pupils

    1. Causes of anisocoria (unequal pupils):

        a. Horner's syndrome: See above.

        b. Third nerve lesion: Unilateral large pupil; also ophthalmoplegia and ptosis. Anisocoria is worse in light (vs. Horner's syndrome).

Pupil involvement suggests compression, because pupillary parasympathetic fibers are the most superficial (vs. ischemic 3rd nerve, often pupil-sparing).

  1) **H&P:** Aneurysm (especially P-comm) > ischemia (e.g. DM or HTN) > trauma, uncal herniation, tumor,.... In an alert pt., a fixed dilated pupil is almost never herniation.
  2) **R/o P-comm aneurysm:** Immediate CT and LP to r/o bleed, consider angiogram.

  c. **Drug effects:**
  1) **Dilators** (mydriatics): Sympathetics, e.g. atropine, scopolamine, phenylephrine, tropicamide, albuterol. Test with 1% pilocarpine (a parasympathetic agonist)—it will <u>not</u> constrict pupil if the pupil was previously drug-dilated, but will in 3rd nerve compression or Adie's syndrome.
  2) **Constrictors:** Parasympathetics, e.g. pilocarpine.

  d. **Acute glaucoma:** Fixed pupil, about 6 mm. Also see red, painful eye, blurred vision, shallow anterior chamber if side-illuminated with penlight.
  1) **Rx:** <u>Emergent</u> IV acetazolamide or mannitol; topical pilocarpine.

  e. **Adie's (tonic) pupil:** One large pupil, reacts poorly to light, with better constriction to near targets; then redilates sluggishly. Often sudden, in young woman, with decreased DTRs.
  1) **Test:** Dilute pilocarpine (0.1%) will constrict Adie's pupil but not normal pupil.

  f. **Argyll-Robertson:** Small irregular unequal (sometimes equal) pupils, constrict to near targets better than light.
  1) **DDx:** syphilis, diabetic pseudo-tabes,....

  g. **Old ocular surgery or trauma.**

  h. **Physiologic anisocoria:** Should be < 1 mm different in both light and dark, briskly reactive.

2. **Causes of bilateral fixed or poorly reactive pupils:**
  a. **Bilateral large pupils:**
  1) **Fixed:** Death, subtotal medullary lesion, immediately postanoxia or hypothermia, severe hypoglycemia, bilateral or nuclear 3rd nerve palsy, botulism.
  2) **Reactive:** Anxiety, opiate withdrawal, aerosolized albuterol, overdose of IV dopamine, atropine, aminoglycosides, tetracycline, Mg, amyl nitrite.

  b. **Midsized pupils:** Dorsal midbrain lesion, e.g. from hydrocephalus. May see sluggish reaction to near, as in Argyll-Robertson pupil.

  c. **Pinpoint pupils:** Opiates, pontine lesion (usually with skew deviation or ophthalmoplegia), metabolic encephalopathy.

3. **Afferent pupillary defect (APD, Marcus-Gunn pupil):** Transient dilation as flashlight moves from good to bad eye. From optic neuritis or retinal lesion.

F. **Vision:** Sudden visual loss is an emergency.
1. **H&P:** Time course of visual loss, eye pain, headache, fevers, joint pain, DM, Check BP, ocular and carotid bruits, fundi (disc pallor, papilledema, retinopathy, arterial occlusion or cholesterol plaque, cherry

red spot), red desaturation, pinhole correction, Amsler grid for meta-
morphopsia, size of blind spot.

    a. Whenever you use dilating drops to examine the fundi, note it
clearly in the chart so the next examiner won't think the pt. is herniating.

2. **Poor acuity:** Suggests eye or optic nerve problem.
3. **Binocular blindness:** Usually from a lesion at the optic chiasm (e.g.
pituitary mass) or in both occipital lobes (e.g. bilateral PCA infarcts),
unless both eyes have been exposed to the same insult.
4. **Monocular blindness:** Transient (TMB) or permanent loss, sudden
and nontraumatic.

    a. Causes:

      1) **TMB:** Embolus or thrombus, often from carotid lesion. 11% of
TMB pts. later have stroke, 41% of them within 1 wk. Temporal arteritis or other vasculitis,....

      2) **Sudden permanent monocular blindness:** All causes of TMB,
plus optic neuritis, intraocular bleed, retinal detachment, acute
angle closure glaucoma, infection,....

    b. Types of retinal infarct:

      1) **Central retinal artery:** Cherry red spot seen in fundus after 6
h.

      2) **Branch retinal artery:** Fundus pallor along that branch.

      3) **Anterior ischemic optic neuropathy:** See papilledema. Often
idiopathic; sometimes arteritis.

    c. Tests: ESR, fibrinogen, TEE, temporal artery biopsy (within days
of starting steroids). See also stroke workup, p. 18

    d. Rx of TMB:

      1) **Prednisone** 60 mg qd until artery biopsy results are back.

      2) **IV heparin:** See p. 127.

      3) **Decrease intraocular pressure:** To help move a possible em-
bolus through the eye. Hypercarbia probably does <u>not</u> help.

        a) **Massage eye:** Have pt. press hard x 4 sec; off x 4 sec.

        b) **IV mannitol** 50 g, or IV acetazolamide 400 mg. Watch BP.

        c) **Anterior paracentesis** by ophthalmologist.

    e. Rx of optic neuritis: See Demyelinating dz, p. 28.

5. **Visual field defects:**

    a. Monocular scotoma: Prechiasmal lesion, e.g. glaucoma, retinal
hemorrhage, optic neuritis, retinal detachment.

    b. Noncongruent bilateral scotomata: Chiasm + nerve lesion.

    c. Bitemporal defect: Chiasmal lesion, e.g. aneurysm or pituitary
mass. Consider glaucoma.

    d. Homonymous defect (same side in both eyes): Postchiasmal.

      1) **Sparing macula:** Visual cortex.

      2) **Including macula:** Optic radiations.

      3) **Superior quadrant defect:** Optic radiations in inferior tempo-
ral lobe, which can be affected by mastoid infection causing
cerebritis

      4) **Inferior quadrant defect:** Optic radiations in parietal lobe.

6. **Higher visual system abnormalities:**

    a. Anton's syndrome: Bilateral occipital lesions cause blindness, but pt. denies he or she is blind.

  b. Bonnet's syndrome: Visual deprivation hallucinations (formed, stereotyped, no other signs of delirium).

  c. Motion and visuospatial processing: Dorsal, occipitoparietal "where" pathway.

    1) **Balint's syndrome:** Visual disorientation (simultanagnosia), optic ataxia (deficit of visual reaching), ocular apraxia (deficit of visual scanning). From bilateral occipitoparietal lesion.

  d. Object recognition (visual agnosia): Ventral, occipitotemporal "what" pathway lesions.

    1) **Prosopagnosia:** Inability to recognize faces; from bilateral inferior visual association cortex lesions.

    2) **Word blindness:** Alexia without agraphia. Seen in left hemisphere lesion near splenium of callosum. Usually with R homonymous hemianopsia and color anomia or achromatopsia.

    3) **Achromatopsia vs. color anomia:** In former, pt. can't perceive colors; in latter he or she can perceive them but not name them.

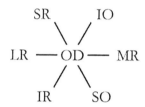

Figure 6. Direction of ocular muscle action, right eye.

G. Eye Movement Abnormalities

  1. See also: Cranial nerves, p. 27.

  2. Acute extraocular paralysis is an emergency: Consider botulism, myasthenic crisis, P-comm aneurysm, cavernous sinus thrombosis, infection, or fistula, variant Guillain-Barré syndrome.

  3. Eye muscles: Figure 6 shows the main field of action of individual eye muscles.

  4. Causes of ophthalmoplegias: Nerve palsy, brainstem lesion, raised ICP with herniation, strabismus, myasthenia gravis, drugs (especially phenytoin), multiple sclerosis, Graves' dz, orbital entrapment, trauma, meningitis or other infection, migraine, Wernicke's syndrome, Fisher variant of GBS, mitochondrial dz.

    a. Causes of painful opthalmoplegias: Cavernous sinus tumor, thrombosis, fistula, or dissection; zoster, DM, migraine, infection.

  5. Diplopia without visibly disconjugate gaze:

    a. H&P: Direction of greatest deficit, h/o lazy eye, drugs, thyroid dz, pain, alteration with fatigue. Note head tilt (compare with old photo), check Bell's reflex, stereopsis, ocular bruit.

    b. Red glass test: Convention is to hold it over R eye. Have pt. report relative positions of red and normal images in all directions of gaze. Diplopia is maximal in the field of gaze of the paretic muscle, and the image belonging to the paretic muscle projects peripherally.

   c. **Alternating cover test:** For phoria (latent): shift cover to other eye while fixating. If covered eye moves in, it's exophoria; if out, it's esophoria, if down, it's hyperphoria; if up, it's hypophoria. If eyes are never conjugate (but not paralyzed), it's a tropia, not a phoria.

6. **Bilateral conjugate gaze palsies:**
   a. **Bilateral fixed eyes:**
      1) **Caloric test:** See p. 189. No response to caloric test suggests brainstem injury. COWS (cold opposite, warm same) gives direction of fast component of nystagmus in an alert person. If coma without brainstem injury, may see only tonic deviation towards cold.
      2) **Doll's eye test:** Do only if C-spine is stable.
   b. **Bilateral upgaze palsy:** The main vertical gaze center is the rostral interstitial nucleus of the medial longitudinal fasciculus (riMLF) in dorsal midbrain; there may be another at the cervicomedullary junction.
      1) **Causes:** Can tell supranuclear lesion (e.g. progressive supranuclear palsy, Parinaud's syndrome) from age-related dystrophy of elevators by presence of other deficits, and by the following tests:
         a) **Bell's reflex:** Eyes normally roll up when pt. tries to close lids against resistance. This reflex is intact in supranuclear lesions.
         b) **Vertical doll's eyes:** Have pt. fix on a target while you move his or her head. Intact in supranuclear lesions.
         c) **Light-near dissociation.** Present in pretectal lesions.
      2) **Parinaud's syndrome:** Dorsal midbrain lesion, e.g. from basilar stroke or pineal tumor. Upgaze worse than downgaze. Often convergence paresis, retraction nystagmus, and lid retraction ("setting sun eyes") on attempted upgaze. May see skew deviation.
   c. **Bilateral downgaze palsy:** Early progressive supranuclear palsy, bilateral ventral midbrain lesions, anoxic coma.
   d. **Bilateral lateral deviation:** Contralateral cerebral hemisphere or midbrain lesion; ipsilateral pons lesion.
      1) **Causes:** Lesion of 6th nucleus, pedunculopontine reticular formation (PPRF), L frontal (in latter, doll's eyes can overcome gaze paresis), parietal neglect.
      2) **Nuclear 6th nerve vs. PPRF lesion:** Central 6th nerve lesion gets 7th nerve as well (genu of VII wraps around nucleus of VI), giving an ipsilateral lower motor neuron 7th palsy (forehead spared). This is not seen in a PPRF lesion.
   e. **Internuclear ophthalmoplegia (INO)**
      1) **H&P:**
         a) **Ipsilateral eye:** Poor adduction to nose.
         b) **Contralateral eye:** Abduction nystagmus (on lateral gaze).
         c) **Convergence:** There is sometimes convergence paresis.

2) **Location:** Lesion is on side of the eye with poor adduction, in the medial longitudinal fasciculus (MLF) , rostral to 6th nerve nucleus (blocks path from 6th to contralateral 3rd nerves), anywhere from pons to midbrain.

3) **DDx:** The elderly usually have vascular causes; young adults usually MS; children usually pontine glioma. Myasthenia can cause a "pseudo-INO."

f. One-and-a-half syndrome: An INO plus horizontal gaze palsy. The ipsilateral eye cannot adduct or abduct. The contralateral eye cannot adduct and has abduction nystagmus. The lesion is lower in the pons than that giving an INO; it is at the level of the 6th nerve nucleus and involves the MLF and PPRF.

g. Congenital progressive external ophthalmoplegia (CPEO): See p. 58.

7. **Skew deviation:** A vertical misalignment, seen in posterior fossa and brainstem lesions.

8. **Unilateral ophthalmoplegia:**

   a. Individual muscle palsy: See Figure 6, p. 39.

   b. CN III (oculomotor): See also Pupils, p. 36.

   1) **H&P:** Fixed and dilated pupil, ptosis. Only lateral gaze is intact, so eye is deviated down and out. Superior trunk controls upgaze and lid; inferior trunk controls downgaze and pupil.

   2) **Causes:** Important to rule out P-comm aneurysm immediately (see p. 37). Midbrain lesion usually has contralateral hemiparesis too. Pupil-sparing palsy suggests nerve ischemia, also temporal arteritis or myasthenia. Often idiopathic.

   c. CN IV (trochlear):

   1) **H&P:** Diplopia on looking down and in. Often compensatory head tilt away from side of lesion. Look at driver's license to see if head tilt is old.

   2) **Bielshowsky's test:** Look for hypertropia and diplopia on straight gaze, R gaze vs. L, and R head tilt vs L tilt.

   3) **Causes:** Closed head trauma > vascular > tumor. Often idiopathic.

   d. CN VI (abducens):

   1) **H&P:** In a nerve lesion only the ipsilateral eye can't look laterally. A nuclear lesion also impairs contralateral eye's ability to look toward the lesioned side.

   2) **Causes:** Tumor (30%) > trauma, ischemic, high ICP, Graves' dz, idiopathic, Wernicke's syndrome,....

   e. Cavernous sinus syndromes

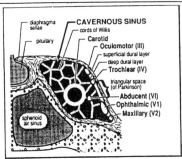

Figure 7. The cavernous sinus. (From Greenberg MS. *Handbook of Neurosurgery*, 3rd ed. Greenberg Graphics, 1994:113, with permission.).

1) **H&P:** Variable involvement of CN III, IV, V$_{1-2}$, VI. An isolated 6th nerve palsy with a Horner's syndrome is a giveaway. Often with pain and proptosis.
2) **DDx:** Carotid artery aneurysm, dissection; venous thrombosis, infection, tumor, Tolosa-Hunt or Wernicke's syndrome,....
3) **Tolosa-Hunt syndrome:** Idiopathic granuloma near the superior orbital fissure, causing pain and CN III, IV, or VI palsies. Responds to steroids. Don't confuse it with Ramsay-Hunt syndrome, p. 73.

9. **Nystagmus:** Nystagmus which is pure, without a mixed rotatory/linear component, is generally of central origin.
   a. H&P: Note whether nystagmus is present in primary gaze; direction of fast component, whether it extinguishes with fixation. Look for accompanying palatal or facial myoclonus, which suggests denervation of the inf. olive, by damage to the central tegmental tract.
   b. Causes: See also Vertigo, p. 98.
      1) **Horizontal:**
         a) **Jerk nystagmus:** Saccadic movement in one direction; slow corrective movement in the other. Causes include drugs, cerebellar or brainstem lesion, vestibular dz, congenital syndromes. A few beats of end-gaze nystagmus may be normal.
         b) **Pendular nystagmus:** Slow movements in both directions. Drugs and vestibular causes are uncommon (unlike jerk nystagmus). Seen in congenital blindness.
      2) **Downbeat:** Often craniocervical junction problem causing anterior cerebellar vermis lesion, e.g. with Chiari malformation. Also MS, drugs, Wernicke's syndrome,....
      3) **Upbeat:** Often medullary lesion; also MS, drugs, Wernicke's...
      4) **Rotatory:** If in combination with horizontal nystagmus and vertigo, usually a peripheral, vestibular lesion. If pure rotatory, usually medullary or diencephalic.

10. **Other ocular oscillations:**

    a. **Square wave jerks:** Small-amplitude macrosaccades on attempted fixation. Causes: often cerebellar or demyelinating dz.

    b. **Ocular bobbing:** Constant, conjugate down-and-up oscillations — fast down, then slow drift back to midposition 2-12 x/min, with horizontal gaze paralysis. Should distinguish it from vertical nystagmus. Causes: Often pontine lesion; sometimes metabolic or from hydrocephalus. Consider also vertical nystagmus.

    c. **Ocular dysmetria:** Eye over- or undershoots target, then makes refixation saccades. Causes: often cerebellar dz. Distinguish from hypometric saccades, in which eye always undershoots; a sign of extrapyramidal bradykinesia.

    d. **Ocular flutter:** Rapid bursts of horizontal oscillations in primary gaze. Similar causes to opsoclonus.

    e. **Opsoclonus:** Continuous, conjugate, multidirectional saccades. Causes: often paraneoplastic syndrome; MS, postviral opsoclonus-myoclonus; encephalitis, drugs, tumors.

HEADACHE

A. H&P: Similarity to previous HAs, onset and time course, N/V, photophobia, neck pain, trauma, fever, neurological aura, change in sx with position, h/o cancer, family history of aneurysms or migraine, what drugs work for pain. Cranial or sinus tenderness, eye changes, focal neurological signs.

B. Causes:

    1. **Sudden paroxysmal headache (HA):** Intracranial hemorrhage (especially subarachnoid), arterial dissection, benign orgasmic HA, thunderclap migraine, hypertensive crisis,....

    2. **Subacute progressive HA:** Posterior fossa stroke, cerebral vein thrombosis, temporal arteritis, tumor, obstructive hydrocephalus, CSF leak, (e.g. post-LP), meningitis, sinusitis, or other infection, vascular malformations, glaucoma,....

    3. **Recurrent or chronic HA:** Migraine, neck arthritis, postconcussive syndrome, pseudotumor cerebri, neuralgia, temporal arteritis, temporomandibular syndrome, drugs (stimulants, solvents, alcohol withdrawal),....

C. Tests:

    1. **Sudden or subacute HA:** CT without contrast to r/o bleed; or with contrast to r/o tumor.

        a. **Consider also:** MRA to r/o vascular malformations, dissections, aneurysm. LP to r/o SAH, meningitis, or leptomeningeal carcinomatosis.

    2. **Recurrent or chronic HA:** Can usually be diagnosed without tests. Consider ESR.

D. Cluster HA:

    1. **H&P:** Nightly, nonthrobbing, uniorbital, ipsilateral running nose, red eye, red cheek, tender temporal artery, lasts 10 min - 2 h, sometimes Horner's syndrome. Alcohol can trigger. Typically youngish men.

    2. **DDx:** Migraine, trigeminal neuralgia, sinus tumor, Tolosa-Hunt,....

    3. **Rx:** Ergot, 100% O_2, methysergide, prednisone taper (can cause re-

bound). Prophylaxis is more effective than treating acute attack; try calcium channel blocker, or lithium.
E. **Post-concussive syndrome:** Try a TCA (see p. 130).
F. **LP HA:** From continued CSF leak. Worse when standing.
   1. **Rx:** Lie flat x 24 h; aggressive fluids (especially carbonated, caffeinated drinks), pain drugs. Consider blood patch, IM steroids, abdominal binder.
G. **HIV HA:** See p. 46.
H. **Occipital neuralgia:** Pain in occiput, usually with trigger point along superior nuchal line. Injection of local anesthetic and steroids may help.
I. **Migraine:**
   1. **H&P:** Unilateral (but not <u>always</u> same side), throbbing, N/V, photophobia, phonophobia, often preceded by visual or other neurologic change.
   2. **Rx of acute migraine:**
      a. **Treat nausea:** e.g. with phenothiazine like metoclopramide 10 mg PO/IM/IV
      b. **Sumatriptan** (Imitrex): $5-HT_1$ serotonin receptor agonist. SC: 6 mg. PO: 25 mg test; if partial relief in 2 h, try up to 100 mg PO; no more than 300 mg qd. Nasal spray 5-20 mg into one nostril, q2h if needed, not more than 40 qd.
         1) **Contraindications:** Ergots within 24 h, possible CAD.
      c. **NSAID:** e.g. naproxen 500 mg PO.
      d. **Ergots:**
         1) **Contraindications:** CAD, HTN, hemiplegic or aphasic migraine (ergots are vasoconstrictors).
         2) **Dihydroergotamine (DHE):** Put patient on a cardiac monitor for first DHE dose. Give metoclopramide 10 mg IV 10 min beforehand; then 1 mg DHE; repeat in 1 h prn; then q6h prn. If it works, try DHE nasal spray, or Cafergot PO.
         3) **Cafergot:** Ergotamine and caffeine. Give 2 tabs, then 1 q30min, max 6 in 24 h.
      e. **Midrin:** A sympathomimetic amine with a sedative. Give 2 tabs, then 1qh to relief; max 5 in 12 h.
         1) **Contraindications:** HTN, glaucoma, renal failure, MAOIs.
      f. **Fioricet:** 1-2 tabs q4h, for attacks fewer than 3x/mo. Beware rebound HA.
      g. **Steroids:** For status migrainosus.
   3. **Prophylaxis of migraine** (if having migraines more than 3x/month):
      a. **Aspirin:** qd for everyone.
      b. **TCAs:** Amitriptyline is the only one with proven efficacy, though nortriptyline is probably also effective, and better tolerated.
      c. **Propranolol:** Start 10-20 bid. Avoid in asthma, CHF.
      d. **5-HT antagonists:** e.g. methysergide. Need test dose. Danger of retroperitoneal fibrosis.
      e. **Calcium blockers:** e.g. verapamil.
      f. **Anticonvulsants:** e.g. valproic acid 250-500 mg tid. See p. 130.
J. **Rebound HAs:** Common after stopping opiates, Fioricet, NSAIDs. Can cause vicious cycle of analgesic use.

HEARING

A. Weber's test: Tuning fork on vertex.
  1. **Conductive (middle ear) deafness:** Fork heard better in affected ear.
  2. **Perceptive (inner ear) deafness:** Fork heard better in good ear.
B. Rinne's test: Tuning fork on mastoid first; when no longer heard, hold it in air by ear.
  1. **Normal:** Air conduction heard twice as long as bone conduction.
  2. **Conductive deafness:** Air conduction briefer than bone conduction.
  3. **Perceptive deafness:** Test is normal (air conduction heard longer.)
C. Causes of deafness:
  1. **Middle ear:** Wax, mass, foreign body, trauma, infection, otosclerosis.
  2. **Cochlea:** Menière's dz, inflammation, trauma, tumor, toxin (aminoglycosides, cisplatin), vasculitis (Cogan's syndrome), internal auditory artery occlusion.
  3. **Retrocochlear:** Cerebellopontine angle mass (acoustic Schwannoma, meningioma, aneurysm, dermoid, epidermoid), multiple sclerosis, brainstem glioma, syringobulbia, inflammation (zoster), brainstem infarct (especially AICA).

INFECTIONS, CNS

A. Abscess and focal cerebritis
  1. **H&P:** Headache, stiff neck, confusion. Focal signs and papilledema are uncommon early. Look for other infections, especially ear, nose, mouth, lung, and heart. Ask about HIV risk factors.
  2. **DDx:** Tumor, granuloma.
  3. **Causes:** Anaerobic streptococci are most common. Posttraumatic or surgical cases are more likely to be staphylococcus or enterobacteriaceae. Many abscesses are polymicrobial.
  4. **Tests:** CT with contrast should show ring-enhancing cavity. Blood cultures, CXR, consider echocardiogram. LP is <u>contraindicated</u>.
  5. **Rx:**
      a. **Surgery:** Needle aspiration or excision of abscess, ideally before Abx initiated.
      b. **Abx:** Treat for 6 wk. Adjust on basis of abscess cultures.
          1) **Ear or unknown source:** penicillin G 5 M U IV q6h + ceftriaxone 2 g IV q12h + metronidazole 500 mg IV q6h.
          2) **HIV-positive:** Add coverage for toxoplasmosis; see below.
          3) **Post-head trauma or surgery:** Replace penicillin with vancomycin 1 g IV q12h.
      c. **Steroids:** Only if severely high ICP, as steroids will decrease antibiotic penetration.
B. Cryptococcosis: A fungus, *Cryptococcus neoformans*. Cryptococcal meningitis <u>may be an emergency</u>, as pts. occasionally die suddenly from high ICP.
  1. **H&P:** HIV, immunosuppression, pigeon exposure. Headache, meningeal signs, confusion, signs of high ICP. Seizures uncommon.
  2. **DDx:** Other meningitides.
  3. **Tests:** CSF (see p. 17). CSF india ink stain is positive in 75%. Serum

cryptococcal Ag. CT usually normal.

    4. Rx: Regimens vary; consider amphotericin B and flucytosine, then fluconazole . Consider serial LPs for high ICP.

C. Cysticercosis: A helminth, the pig tapeworm *Taenia solis.*

    1. H&P: Country of origin, seizures, headache, signs of raised ICP.

    2. DDx: Other parasitic dz.

    3. Tests: Stool ova and parasites. Blood serology better than CSF; but slow. Consider long bone X-ray series to look for calcified muscle cysts.

    4. Rx: Albendazole 15 mg/kg qd for 8 d. Give with steroids because dying cysts cause inflammation. Consider surgery for posterior fossa or intraventricular cysts. If cysts are inactive, may not need to treat. Treat seizures.

        a. Rule out macular cysts prior to albendazole (check acuity and fundi).

        b. Ventricular cysts: Consider surgery.

D. Empyema, CNS: An <u>immediate surgical emergency</u>. Usually see pain out of proportion to neurological deficit.

    1. Brain subdural empyemas: Frequently from sinusitis or trauma. Unlike subdural blood, they are better seen on MRI than CT. Consult ENT preoperatively for sinus drainage during the same procedure. Watch for sinus thrombosis.

    2. Spinal cord empyemas: Never do an LP in a pt. with fever and back pain until you have ruled out empyema with MRI.

E. Human immunodeficiency virus (HIV): See also Infections, p. 176.

    1. Incidence: 50% of HIV pts. have a CNS or PNS problem; this can be the presenting complaint.

    2. Headache: Have a very low threshold for CT + contrast and LP. All pts. with HA and fever should get both.

    3. Focal brain sx: Consider toxoplasmosis, lymphoma, progressive multifocal leukoencephalopathy (PML), cryptococcus, VZV encephalitis, tuberculoma, neurosyphilis, clot, bleed, bacterial abscess.

    4. Nonfocal/encephalitic sx:

        a. HIV dementia complex: Subcortical dementia with psychomotor slowing; often frontal, extrapyramidal, or pyramidal signs.

        b. Encephalitis: CMV, HSV, HIV.

        c. Metabolic encephalopathies.

    5. Meningeal sx: Meningitis from HIV (primary infection), cryptococcus, TB, syphilis, bacterial, lymphomatous.

    6. Cranial neuropathies: CNS lesion, meningitis, peripheral neuropathy.

    7. Spinal cord sx: B_{12} deficiency, HTLV-1, HSV or VZV myelitis; vacuolar myelopathy.

    8. Peripheral nerve sx: Can be immune-mediated, drug-induced (e.g. didanosine [ddI], zalcitabine[ddC], or Kaposi's chemotherapy), or infectious (e.g. CMV or VZV radiculopathy).

        a. Lumbosacral polyradiculopathy (cauda equina syndrome): Subacute leg weakness ± back pain, early bowel and bladder problems.

      1) **DDx:** Usually CMV. Consider also lymphomatous meningitis, neurosyphilis, spinal cord mass.

      2) **Tests:** LP shows > 500 WBCs/μl (often with high PMNs), high protein, normal or low glucose. EMG shows axonal and demyelinating lesion,....

      3) **Rx of lumbosacral polyradiculopathy:** Ganciclovir or foscarnet.

   9. **Myopathy:** From zidovudine (AZT)

F. Lyme dz:

   1. **H&P:**

     a. **Early** (3 d-1 mo): Erythema migrans in ~70%, flu-like sx.

     b. **Middle** (up to 9 mo): Recurrent meningitis, radiculo- and cranial neuritis (especially peripheral 7th nerve), arthralgias.

     c. **Late:** Mild encephalopathy, MS-like lesions on MRI, seizures.

   2. **Tests:** CSF Lyme Ab titer (only test CSF if seropositive).

   3. **Rx:**

     a. **Isolated 7th nerve palsy or mild neuropathy:** e.g. amoxicillin 1 g PO q6h + probenecid 500 mg q6h x 30 d. An alternate is doxycycline 100 mg tid x 30 d.

     b. **More serious neurological sx:** Ceftriaxone 2 g IV qid x 2-6 wk.

G. Meningitis

   1. **Bacterial meningitis is an emergency:** It may be necessary to give IV Abx empirically before the LP. LP can be done up to 2 h after first dose without destroying culture results.

   2. **H&P:** Prior focal signs, earache, cough, gastroenteritis, immunosuppression, trauma. Temperature, rash, photophobia, fundi, stiff neck, oto- or rhinorrhea.

     a. **Brudzinski's sign:** Bending chin to chest makes hips and knees flex.

     b. **Kernig's sign:** Pain on straight leg raise. Could also be nerve compression.

   3. **Tests:** CT (consider contrast), LP (see p. 191, and see Cerebrospinal fluic, p. 17), blood cultures, CBC, HIV test, CXR. Consider testing nasal discharge for glucose, chloride to r/o CSF leak.

   4. **DDx of meningitis:** Tumor + fever, abscess, toxic exposure,...

   5. **Bacterial meningitis:**

Patient	Likely pathogen	Antibiotic
Immunocompetent		
18-50 yrs	*S. pneumoniae* or *N. meningitidis*	Ceftriaxone 2 g IV q12h + vancomycin 500 mg IV q6h
>50 yrs	*S. pneumoniae.*, *L. monocytogenes*, or gram-negative bacilli	Ampi. 2 g IV q4h + ceftriaxone 2 g IV q 2h + vanco. 500 mg IV q6h
Immunocompromised	*L. monocytogenes*, gram-negative bacilli	Ampicillin 2 g IV q4h + ceftazidime 50-100 mg/kg IV q8h
Head trauma, surgery, or shunt	Staphylococci, gram-negative bacilli, or *S. pneumoniae*	Vancomycin 15 mg/kg IV q6h + ceftazidime 50-100 mg/kg IV q8h

Table 7. Empiric antibiotics for bacterial meningitis. Adjust on basis of C+S. (Adapted from Quagliarello VJ, Sheld WM. N Engl J Med. 1997;336:708,with permission.)

     a. **Orders:** Droplet precautions if danger of meningococcus. If there is high ICP, give dexamethasone 0.15 mg/kg IV q6h x 4d.

6. **Viral meningoencephalitis:**
    a. **Herpes simplex encephalitis:**
        1) **HSV encephalitis is an emergency:** Acyclovir should be started empirically, before HSV PCR is back.
        2) **H&P:** Viral prodrome; then rapid progression of floridly abnormal behavior, amnesia, seizures, hemiplegia, coma.
        3) **Tests:** HSV PCR in CSF; high CSF RBCs, monos, and protein. MRI may show ant. temporal lobe edema, uncal herniation. EEG shows periodic lateralized epileptiform discharges.
        4) **Rx:** Acyclovir 10 mg/kg IV q8h for 7-10 d. Watch closely for signs of uncal transtentorial herniation.
    b. **Others:** Varicella, enterovirus, mumps, arboviruses (e.g. eastern equine encephalitis, St. Louis encephalitis), rabies.

7. **Tuberculous meningitis and tuberculomas:**
    a. **H&P:** Recent TB exposure, HIV risk factors. Slow onset of headache, low-grade fever, then meningismus and focal neurological signs. In young pts. but not in secondary reactivation, it is usually associated with disseminated dz.
    b. **Tests:** CSF shows lymphocytosis, low glucose, high protein, and positive AFB cultures (after 4-6 wk). AFB stain is frequently negative. PPD is negative in 1/3 of pts. CXR shows pulmonary TB in about 75%.
    c. **Rx:** If suspicious, must start rx before CSF cultures come back. Check with a specialist for current recommendations, but typical practice starts with isoniazid, rifampin, pyrazinamide, and ethambutol. Give pyridoxine supplements; watch for hypersensitivity, liver dysfunction, and neuropathy. Steroids are sometimes used if there is high ICP, encephalopathy, or evidence of vasculitis.

8. **Chronic or recurrent meningitis**
    a. **DDx of chronic meningitis:**
        1) **Noninfectious:** Neoplasm, sarcoid, vasculitis, lupus, Vogt-Koyanagi-Harada syndrome, Behçet's dz, chronic benign lymphocytic meningitis, Mollaret's meningitis, chemical meningitis, post-SAH,....
        2) **Infectious:** TB, fungal, cysticercosis, HACEK organisms, Lyme, brucellosis, syphilis.
    b. **Tests:**
        1) **Blood:**
            a) **General:** Electrolytes, LFTs, CBC, ESR, ANA, RF, ACE, SIEP, VDRL.
            b) **Antibodies:** to *Brucella*, toxoplasmosis, cryptococcus, Lyme, histoplasmosis, coccidiomycosis.
            c) **Antigens:** Cryptococcus.
        2) **CSF:**
            a) **Cultures:** Bacterial, mycobacterial, fungal cultures. Consider volume.> 10 ml; prolonged (HACEK organisms), CO_2 (*Brucella*), or anerobic (*Actinomyces*) incubations.
            b) **Assays:** Cryptococcal Ag and Ab, India ink prep for fungi, AFB, VDRL.
            c) **Cytology:** Mollaret's cells, flow cytometry.

3) **Imaging:** MRI for parameningeal abscess; consider CXR, spine, skull films.
4) **Other:** PPD, sputum AFB, stool fungi, meningeal biopsy.

H. Progressive multifocal leukoencephalopathy (PML): Widespread demyelination causes neurological sx over days to weeks. From JC virus infection; usually associated with HIV infection.

I. Syphilis: A spirochete, *Treponema pallidum.*

1. **H&P:** Other sexually transmitted dz, genital lesions, HIV.
   a. **Early meningitis:** 6-12 mo after primary infection.
   b. **Meningovascular:** Cranial neuropathies, especially 7th and 8th nerves, arteritis, stroke.
   c. **Tabes dorsalis:** Sharp leg pains, Argyll-Robertson pupils, proprioceptive ataxia, overflow incontinence, dropped reflexes.
   d. **General paresis of the insane:** May present as almost any psychiatric disorder. Sx of tabes and meningovascular syphilis are uncommon. Often see brisk DTRs, expressionless face, intention tremor.
2. **DDx:** Cryptococccal, TB, or carcinomatous meningitis, CNS sarcoid, Lyme, vasculitis.
3. **Tests:** Serum fluorescent treponemal absorption test positive in 90%. RPR and serum VDRL may be negative. CSF VDRL nearly always positive, with high protein and lymphocytes. HIV test.
4. **Rx:** 24 MU penicillin G IV + 2 g probenecid qd x 21 days.

J. Toxoplasmosis: An intracellular protozoan, *Toxoplasma gondii.*

1. **H&P:** Immunosuppression, focal deficits, headache, confusion, fever, seizures.
2. **DDx:** Lymphoma, bacterial abscess, viral or fungal encephalitis, PML.
3. **Tests:** CT—single or multiple enhancing (usually ring) lesions, with edema. CSF (see p. 17). Toxoplasmosis titer (Ab not useful). HIV test, CD4 count.
4. **Rx:** Acutely, pyrimethamine 200 mg PO x 1; then 100 qd, + folinic acid (not folic) 10 mg PO qd, and sulfadiazine 1 g PO q6h or clindamycin 300 mg PO q6h. For maintenance, lower doses of Abx to 25%.

K. Inflammatory disorders of unknown cause:

1. **Behçet's dz:** Recurrent mouth and genital ulcers, uveitis, skin lesions (erythema nodosum and acneiform rash), and hyperirritability. 25% develop aseptic meningitis; CNS symptoms are occasionally seen.
   a. **Tests:** The pathergy test (formation of a sterile pustule at the site of a pin-prick) is not very specific.
   b. **Rx:** Usually steroids.
2. **Sarcoid:** A granulomatous dz, primarily of lungs. 5% of pts. have neurological involvement.
   a. **Neurological manifestations:** Aseptic meningitis is most common; see also intraparenchymal mass lesion, multifocal white matter dz, vasculopathy, spinal cord or peripheral nerve lesions, myopathy.
   b. **Tests:** CXR, serum calcium, ACE (not very specific), consider gallium scan.

    c. Rx: Usually steroids.
   3. Vogt-Koyanagi-Harada syndrome: Recurrent uveitis, meningoencephalitis, deafness, vitiligo, and hair changes. Usually benign course.

INSTANT NEUROLOGIST

	Focal	Diffuse
Acute	Vascular	Metabolic
Subacute	Inflammatory	Inflammatory
Chronic	Tumor	Degenerative

Table 8. Instant neurological diagnosis.

INTRACRANIAL HEMORRHAGE

A. See also: CT signs of intracranial hemorrhage, p. 145; arterial diagrams in cerebrovascular ischemia, p. 18.

B. Epidural hematoma:
   1. H&P: Classic presentation is trauma with brief loss of consciousness; then lucid interval, then obtundation, contralateral hemiparesis, and ipsilateral pupil dilation.
   2. Rx: <u>Emergency surgery.</u>

C. Subdural hematoma (SDH):
   1. DDx: Epidural hematoma, subdural empyema, cerebral atrophy.
   2. Causes
     a. Acute SDH usually follows trauma.
     b. Chronic spontaneous SDH can be seen in the elderly, especially with cerebral atrophy, alcoholism, epilepsy.
   3. Rx of SDH:
     a. Symptomatic SDH should be surgically drained.
     b. Asymptomatic SDH may be watched.
     c. Seizure prophylaxis.

D. Subarachnoid hemorrhage (SAH): <u>Nontraumatic SAH is an emergency; usually requires immediate angiogram.</u>
   1. H&P: Spontaneous SAH often presents with sudden, severe headache —"the worst HA in my life." N/V, syncope, meningismus, cranial nerve deficits (especially 3rd nerve), obtundation, ocular hemorrhage.
   2. Causes of SAH:
     a. Trauma. Most SAHs are traumatic. However, make sure head trauma preceded LOC, not vice versa.
     b. Aneurysms: 75% of spontaneous SAHs are ruptured aneurysms.
       1) **Location:** 30% A-comm, 25% P-comm, 20% MCA, 10% basilar, 5% vertebral, 25% have multiple aneurysms.
       2) **Associations with aneurysms:** Polycystic kidney dz, fibromuscular dysplasia, AVMs, Ehlers-Danlos syndrome type IV, aortic coarctation, Marfan's or Osler-Weber-Rendu syndrome.
     c. Idiopathic: 15% of spontaneous SAH; associated with cigarettes, oral contraceptives, HTN, EtOH.
     d. Other: AVMs, vasculitis, carotid artery dissection.
   3. Hunt-Hess grading scale in SAH:

0: Unruptured aneurysm.

1: Asymptomatic or mild HA and nuchal rigidity.

2: Moderate or severe HA, nuchal rigidity, ± cranial nerve palsy, e.g. III, VI.

3: Mild focal deficit, lethargy, or confusion.

4: Stupor, moderate/severe hemiparesis, early decerebrate rigidity.

5: Deep coma, decerebrate rigidity, moribund appearance.

4. **Prognosis in SAH:**

   a. **Mortality:** 30% die before reaching hospital; then 10% in first few days, 50% first month.

   b. **Morbidity:** 50-60% have serious deficit even with successful clipping.

   c. **Rebleeding risk:** With unclipped aneurysm, 15% rebleed in 14 days, 50% in 6 mo, then 3%/yr. Hypertension greatly increases rebleed risk.

5. **Tests in SAH:**

   a. **Blood:** PT, PTT, blood bank sample with 6 U held for OR, phenytoin level if pt. has been loaded.

   b. **EKG:** For arrhythmia, MI, cerebral Ts, long QT, U waves.

   c. **CT:** See p. 145 for CT appearance.

   d. **LP:** If negative CT. See high opening pressure, blood that doesn't clear in successive tubes, xanthochromia if bleed > 6 h. WBC may be secondarily elevated.

   e. **Emergent angiogram:** For spontaneous SAH, to r/o correctable aneurysm. Consider calling angiographers to prepare them when you first know of patient. Don't angiogram patients with H-H grade IV-V, because their prognosis is so poor. Reconsider it if pt. improves after ventriculostomy.

      1) **Angiogram-negative spontaneous SAH:** Repeat angio in 2 wk.

6. **Rx of SAH:**

   a. **Immediate SBP control** < 140, usually with nipride. If pt. also having MI, consider nitroglycerine +/- labetalol. Once BP stable, to wean IV agents, start PO β-blocker; add α–block if needed.

   b. **Oxygenation:** If needed for airway protection, intubate after baseline exam. All other patients should get supplementary oxygen.

   c. **Monitoring:** Cardiac monitor, probably arterial and central line, neuro checks q1h, ABG, electrolytes, and CBC qd. Daily CXR, until stable, to r/o neurogenic pulmonary edema.

   d. **Avoid all anticoagulants.**

   e. **Vasospasm prophylaxis:** Nimodipine 60 mg q4h PO x 21 d, gentle volume expansion (e.g. D5 NS +20 KCl at 100 ml/h), but not at expense of keeping SBP low.

   f. **Seizure prophylaxis:** Phenytoin load 1 g; then 100 mg tid. Side effects of phenytoin, e.g. abnormal eye movements, may complicate following the neurological exam.

   g. **ICU orders:** Bedrest with head of bed > 30 degrees, pain drugs, compression hose and airboots, stool softener. Minimize stimulation.

   h. **Hydrocephalus:** Mannitol 50-100 g IV, then 25 q6 for osms <

305-310. Consider ventriculostomy. Beware lowering intracranial pressure quickly; it can cause rebleeding.

i. Dexamethasone: 4-10 mg IV x 1 on call to OR, or for headache

j. Hyponatremia:
  1) **Cause:** Usually cerebral salt wasting (see p. 160), <u>not</u> SIADH.
  2) **Rx:** Gentle volume expansion and salt.

k. Ocular hemorrhage: Consult ophthalmology to follow intraocular pressures.

l. Vasospasm:
  1) **Signs of vasospasm:** Delayed ischemic neurological deficit, usually day 6-8.
  2) **Labs:** ABG to r/o hypoxia, electrolytes to r/o low Na, stat head CT, bedside transcranial ultrasound.
  3) **Rx of SAH-induced vasospasm:** triple-H therapy (hypertension, hypervolemia, and hemodilution).
    a) **Contraindications:** Unclipped aneurysm, severe edema or infarct.
    b) **Hypertensive therapy:** Arterial line, blood/colloid (keep Hct < 40%), then neosynephrine, then fludrocortisone 2 mg qd.
    c) **Other:** Oxygen, consider ICP monitor, dexamethasone 6 mg q6h, bid serum and urine electrolytes.

E. Intracerebral hemorrhage (ICH):

1. **Causes:** Location is guide to cause; see CT signs of ICH, p. 145. Trauma, hypertensive hemorrhage, and amyloid angiopathy are most common causes. But consider also aneurysm, AVM, cavernous malformation, cocaine abuse, tumor, coagulopathy, vasculitis, vasculopathy, e.g. moya-moya dz,....

2. **DDx:** Hemorrhagic transformation of infarct, venous thrombosis, infection (especially endocarditic embolus, fungal, granulomatous, or HSV).
   a. Hemorrhagic transformation of infarct:

	Hemorrhagic infarct	ICH
Symptoms	Max. at onset	Progressive
CT appearance	Blood mottled	Dense, homogeneous
Onset of blood	Often days-weeks after stroke	At time of first deficit
Mass effect	Prominent	Usually minimal

Table 9. Distinguishing hemorrhagic infarct from ICH.

3. **Rx of ICH:**
   a. SBP control: Goal ~140-160. Avoid hypotension if there is significant edema or hydrocephalus.
   b. DVT prophylaxis: Pneumoboots (after leg ultrasounds if in hospital > 24 h); can use SQ heparin in a few days.
   c. Seizure prophylaxis: Controversial; not necessary for noncortical bleeds.
   d. Steroids: Not much effect on swelling from hemorrhage.
   e. Follow-up scan: Consider early (< 2 days) to r/o underlying mass before granulation tissue forms. Consider iron susceptibility se-

quence for prior bleeds. CT + contrast for follow-up after bleed
completely resolved.

  f. Indications for neurosurgery: Depends on estimate of permanent
  disability; desires of pt. Consider decompression or ventriculostomy in acutely deteriorating pt., especially with posterior fossa
  bleeds > 3 cm, secondary hydrocephalus, blood in ventricles
  (which can cause rapid hydrocephalus).

F. Vascular malformations
  1. Arteriovenous malformations: Congenital direct connection between arteries and veins.
    a. H&P: Hemorrhage (~4%/yr; rarely associated with early rebleed-
    ing or vasospasm), seizures, headache, focal deficits, cranial bruits.
    b. Tests: May be seen on MRI or MRA, but arteriogram is needed to
    characterize an AVM's blood supply.
    c. Rx: Endovascular embolization, XRT, or surgery.
  2. Venous angiomas: No arterial inputs. Lower bleed risk than with
  AVMs. Usually seen on MRI.
  3. Cavernous malformations: Sinusoidal vessels without intervening
  neural tissue. Often not seen on angiogram, because of low flow and
  presence of thrombosis.
G. Intraventricular hemorrhage: Usually hypertensive; consider also
  AVM, aneurysm. Pt. will usually need a ventriculostomy.

INTRACRANIAL PRESSURE

A. See also: CT appearance of herniation, p. 147.
B. Sx and progression of herniation:
  1. Central supratentorial herniation: Usually subacute, from tumor.
  Diencephalon is forced down through tentorium.
    a. Diencephalic stage (reversible): Small pupils with light-near dis-
    sociation, roving eyes with decreased upgaze, obtundation, yawn-
    ing. Progresses to Cheyne-Stokes breathing and decorticate pos-
    ture.
    b. Pontine stage (not reversible): Midsized fixed pupils (even though
    pontine lesions cause pinpoint nonreactive pupils). Cheyne-Stokes
    progresses to tachypnea. Decreased doll's eyes and calorics. Dis-
    conjugate gaze ± intranuclear ophthalmoplegia. Decorticate pos-
    ture becomes decerebrate, then flaccid.
    c. Medullary stage: Dilated pupils. Slow, irregular respirations.
  2. Uncal supratentorial herniation: Usually rapid, often from hematoma of temporal lobe.
    a. First stage: Unilateral pupil dilation often before mental status
    change. Uncal herniation can pinch off PCAs.
    b. Second stage: Ophthalmoplegia and hyperventilation. May see
    Kernohan's false localizing sign: ipsilateral hemiplegia as contra-
    lateral peduncle is compressed.
    c. Third stage: Midposition pupils and decerebrate posture.
    d. Fourth stage: Sx of central herniation (see above).
  3. Cingulate herniation.
  4. Subtentorial herniation: Often presents with respiratory arrest, so

prophylaxis is more useful than monitoring.
- **a. Upward cerebellar herniation:** Sometimes see dorsal midbrain syndrome.
- **b. Tonsillar herniation.** Compresses medulla.

C. Causes of high ICP:
1. **Mass lesion:** e.g. blood, tumor, trauma.
2. **Obstruction:** Of CSF flow or resorption.
3. **Cerebral edema:**
   - **a. Vasogenic:** From tumor, abscess. Give steroids.
   - **b. Ischemic:** From stroke, trauma. Give mannitol.
   - **c. Granulocytic:** From infection. Give Abx; steroids are controversial.
   - **d. Interstitial:** From obstructive hydrocephalus.
4. **Pseudotumor cerebri:** (benign intracranial hypertension).
   - **a. H&P:** Headache, papilledema, constricted visual fields. More common in obese women.
   - **b. Causes:** Steroid use, hyper-/hypovitaminosis A, drugs (tetracycline, nitrofurantoin, isotretinoin [Accutane]), anemia.
   - **c. DDx:** Dural sinus thrombosis, mass lesion, meningitis, inflammation (SLE, sarcoid, Behçet's dz).
   - **d. Rx:** Acetazolamide 250-1000 mg PO qd-tid (check electrolytes); repeated LPs weight loss. Periodic checks of visual fields. Consider VP shunt.

D. Tests to assess ICP:
1. **CT:** See p. 146, for CT appearance of high ICP.
2. **CSF pressure:**
   - **a. Methods:** Ventriculostomy allows pressure measurements as well as CSF drainage. ICP monitor (AKA bolt, subarachnoid screw) allows only pressure measurements. LP is <u>contraindicated</u> if you suspect high ICP from mass lesion.
   - **b. Values:** Normal < 7 mm Hg (100 mm water). Needs rx if > 18 mm Hg (200 mm water). Life-threatening if > 25 mm Hg (350 mm water) and mean arterial pressure < 85.
   - **c. Conversions:** 1 mm water = 0.07 mm Hg.
   - **d. Cerebral perfusion pressure** = (mean arterial pressure) - (intracranial pressure).

E. Rx of high ICP:
1. **Mannitol:** 25-100 g (not mg) IV bolus for average-sized person (0.25-1 g/kg). Then 25-50 g q4h for osms < 305-310.
   - **a. Contraindications:** Low BP. Rebound is rare —never use rebound as a reason not to give mannitol. If there is a large volume of damaged blood-brain barrier, there is little effect from mannitol.
   - **b. To discontinue mannitol:** Typical taper is 25 g q6h x 1 d, 25 g q8h x 1 d, 25 g q12h x 1 d, 2 g 5 q24h x 1 d, then stop.
2. **Dexamethasone:** If high ICP is from tumor. 10 mg IV, then 4 q6h.
3. **Hyperventilation:** Last-ditch, temporary effect. Keep pCO_2 ~30.
   - **a. Danger of ischemia:** pH > 7.5 transiently decreases cerebral blood flow through vasoconstriction.
   - **b. Danger of rebound:** Can occur when you raise pCO_2 after pH has compensated, so wean slowly (increase pCO_2 range by 5 U q8h).

4. **Miscellaneous:** HOB up 30 degrees, airboots or SQ heparin.
5. **Avoid:** Nitroprusside, nitroglycerine, and Ca channel blockers, which raise ICP via vasodilation, and therefore decrease cerebral perfusion. Instead use β-blockers or ACE-I for BP control.
6. **Surgery:** e.g. ventriculostomy, ventriculoperitoneal shunt, hemicraniectomy. See p. 67, for decompression techniques.
7. **Barbiturates:** Lower ICP more than BP, so can increase cerebral perfusion. May need pressors. Lower cerebral metabolism.

METABOLIC, TOXIC, AND DEFICIENCY DISORDERS

A. **Metabolic disorders:**
  1. **Electrolyte disorders:** See p. 158.
  2. **Glucose disorders:** See p. 162.
  3. **Hepatic encephalopathy:** See p. 165.
  4. **Thyroid disorders:** See p. 163.
  5. **Uremic encephalopathy:** See p. 182.
B. **Drugs:** See entries in DRUGS, p. 123.
  1. **Alcohol:**
    a. **Dependence:** Consider it especially in patients with depression, unexplained neuropathy, frequent falls, liver abnormalities. CAGE questions: Have you ever thought about Cutting down on your drinking? Do you ever feel Angry when people ask about it? Does it make you feel Guilty? Do you ever have an Eye-opener? Talk to pt. and family members separately; assess impact on job, etc.
    b. **Withdrawal:**
      1) **H&P:** Time of last drink, h/o withdrawal and non-withdrawal seizures, detoxification programs. Tremulousness, tachycardia, orthostatic hypotension, seizures. Focal seizures are rarely alcoholic —does the pt. have a h/o head injuries?
      2) **Tests:** Electrolytes, Ca/Mg/phos, CBC, PT, PTT, LFTs, B_{12}.
      3) **Seizure rx:**
        a) **Acute:** Diazepam 5-10 mg IV, or lorazepam 1-2 mg if pt. has liver dz or if drug must be given IM.
        b) **Chronic:** Dilantin is less helpful, except if patient has a nonalcoholic seizure disorder too.
      4) **Withdrawal prophylaxis:**
        a) **Oxazepam:** 15-30 PO q4-6h or chlordiazepoxide (avoid in liver dz) 25-100 q4h; taper ~20% qd.
        b) **β-Blocker** or clonidine if pt. is actively withdrawing.
        c) **Replete KCl;** Calcium, phosphorus, magnesium.
        d) **Vitamins:** Thiamine 100 mg IM/IV qd, folate 1 mg qd, multivitamin.
        e) **GI prophylaxis:** Ranitidine or sucralfate.
        f) **IV fluids:** D5 1/2 NS + KCl at 150 ml/h.
      5) **Orders:** Guaiac all stools, BP q4h.
    c. **Delirium tremens:** Severe withdrawal. 5-10% mortality. autonomic instability (tachycardia, HTN, sweating, fever); hallucinations, seizures, tremor.
    d. **Wernicke's syndrome:** See p. 57.

    e. Hepatic encephalopathy: See p. 165.

    f. Alcoholic cerebellar degeneration: Truncal ataxia evolves over weeks or months. Nystagmus and limb ataxia are rarer. CT shows vermis atrophy.

    g. Alcoholic neuropathy: Sensory > motor neuropathy, often painful. Vibration sense is lost first.

    h. Marchiafava-Bignami dz: Corpus callosum degeneration, associated with red wine consumption. Presents as a frontal lobe dementia.

    i. Tobacco-alcohol amblyopia: Bilateral optic neuropathy that may progress to blindness over a few weeks. Treat with B vitamins.

  2. Intravenous drugs: Neurological complications of IV use include

    a. Cerebral complications of endocarditis: Abscess, mycotic aneurysm, bacterial meningitis.

    b. Neuropathies: Mononeuropathy 2-3 h after injection, various polyneuropathies and Guillain-Barré syndrome.

    c. Transverse myelitis: Often with reuse after 1-6 mo abstinence; mechanism unclear.

    d. Toxic amblyopia: Probably from quinine contamination.

  3. Opiates: See opiate side effects, p. 125.

  4. Stimulants: e.g. cocaine, amphetamines.

    a. Direct effects: Agitation, progressing to motor stereotypy, psychosis, seizures, coma, malignant hyperthermia, death.

    b. Vascular effects: Cerebral bleeds. Occasionally ischemic stroke in intranasal but not IV users. Small-vessel cerebral vasculitis from cocaine; multiorgan necrotizing vasculitis (like polyarteritis nodosa) from amphetamines.

C. Exogenous toxins:

  1. Carbon monoxide:

    a. H&P: Exposure; HA, N/V, confusion —cherry-red lips, cyanosis, and retinal hemorrhages are rare. Delayed neuropsychiatric sx in 10-30%, resolve after a year in 50-75%.

    b. Rx: 100% O_2. For coma, persistent sx, or pregnant women, consider hyperbaric O_2.

  2. Heavy metals: Arsenic, lead, mercury, and thallium poisoning produce neuropathy. Large doses of other metals can cause neuropathy, but usually systemic signs predominate.

	Exposure	Symptoms
Arsenic	Insecticide, Paris green	Sensory > motor neuropathy, red hands, burning feet, hyperhidrosis
Lead	Paint, gas, batteries	Adults: neuropathy; painful joints. Children: cerebral edema, encephalopathy, low IQ
Mercury	Industrial, polluted fish	Severe arm and leg pain, dementia with primarily motor neuropathy
Thallium	Insecticide, rat poison	Stocking-glove sensorimotor neuropathy, with alopecia

Table 10. Heavy metal toxicity.

    a. Tests: 24-h-urine analysis; blood lead levels.

      b. Rx: For arsenic, lead, or mercury use penicillamine 250 mg PO qid; for thallium, diphenylthiocarbazone or sodium dicarbamate.
  3. Organophosphates: In pesticides, flame retardants. Depressed levels of RBC acetylcholinesterase indicate recent exposure.
      a. Acute effects: Respiratory and neck weakness, up to 2 wk.
      b. Delayed effects: May see central-peripheral axonopathy 1-3 wk after exposure, with paresthesias, distal to proximal weakness.
D. Nutritional syndromes:

Sign	Deficiency
Encephalopathy	B_{12}, folate, nicotinic acid, thiamine
Seizures	Pyridoxine
Myelopathy	B_{12}, folate, vitamin E
Myopathy	Vitamin D, E
Neuropathy	Thiamine, B_{12}, folate, vitamin E, pyridoxine
Optic neuropathy	B_{12}, folate, thiamine, other B vitamins

Table 11. Neurological signs of vitamin deficiency.

  1. Vitamin A: Deficiency causes night blindness and optic atrophy. Excess > 50,000 IU qd causes pseudotumor cerebri.
  2. Thiamine (B_1) deficiency:
    a. Wernicke's syndrome:
      1) **H&P:** Most common in alcoholics, poor nutrition, hyperemesis. Onset may be subacute or acute. See ophthalmoplegia (often bilateral 6th nerve palsy, nystagmus), confusion, truncal ataxia, sometimes signs of alcohol withdrawal.
      2) **Rx:** Thiamine 100 mg IM/IV x 5 d, then PO. Avoid glucose until the first dose of thiamine is given.
      3) **Prognosis:** Death, if untreated. Rx should cause ocular abnormalities to resolve within hours to days; confusion may take days to weeks; ataxia, months. Pt. may be left with Korsakoff's syndrome: anterograde and retrograde amnesia with prominent confabulation, but retained attention and social behavior.
    b. Beriberi: Rare in developed countries. See sensorimotor polyneuropathy, and cardiomyopathy.
  3. Pyridoxine (B_6): In adults, both excess (>500 mg qd for several wk) and deficiency causes peripheral neuropathy. Deficiency is usually from isoniazid, hydralazine, or penicillamine. Some infants are genetically pyridoxine-dependent and require high doses to prevent seizures.
  4. Vitamin B_{12} deficiency:
    a. H&P: h/o malabsorption, anemia. Distal paresthesias, then weak, unsteady gait are the most common presentations, but confusion, psychiatric sx, or visual impairment are sometimes seen first. Exam shows polyneuropathy, myelopathy, or both. There may be central scotomata, brainstem, or cerebellar signs.
    b. Tests: Macrocytic anemia is not always present. B_{12} levels are usually low, but perform a Schilling test for pernicious anemia if suspicion is high, even if B_{12} levels are normal.
    c. Rx: B_{12} 100 μcg IM qd x 2 wk, then 1000 μcg qwk x 2 mo, then

1000 μcg IM qmo. There is new evidence that oral B_{12}, 1000 μcg BID, may be as well absorbed as IM, even in pernicious anemia. Do not give folate until B_{12} has been repleted for 1-2 wk.

5. **Vitamin E deficiency:** Often from fat malabsorption. See spinocerebellar degeneration, often with peripheral neuropathy, sometimes pigmentary retinopathy, nystagmus, ophthalmoplegia, and proximal weakness.

6. **Folate deficiency:** In alcoholism, pregnancy, phenytoin use. Can cause B_{12}-like syndrome but not dementia. In first trimester of pregnancy, causes spina bifida.

MITOCHONDRIAL DISORDERS

A. **Tests:** Blood lactate, more sensitive after a glucose load or during a crisis. Muscle biopsy. Mitochondrial DNA analysis.

B. **Kearns-Sayre syndrome (KSS):** AKA congenital progressive external ophthalmoplegia (CPEO). See Table 12.

C. **Leber's hereditary optic neuropathy:** Progressive blindness from optic atrophy.

D. **Leigh's dz** (subacute necrotizing encephalomyelopathy): Usually pediatric, with hypotonia, developmental delay, apneic episodes; sometimes seizures, ataxia, neuropathy, ophthalmoplegia.

E. **Myoclonic epilepsy with ragged red fibers (MERRF):** See Table 12.

F. **Mitochondrial encephalopathy with lactic acidosis and stroke-like episodes (MELAS):** See Table 12.

G. **Neuropathy, ataxia, and retinitis pigmentosa:** Also see growth retardation, dementia.

	KSS	MERRF	MELAS
Weakness	±	+	+
Ragged red fibers	+	+	+
Short stature	+	+	+
Deafness	+	+	+
Dementia	+	+	+
Spongy brain degeneration	+	+	+
Ophthalmoplegia	+		
Retinal degeneration	+		
Heart block	+		
CSF protein > 100 mg/dl	+		
Myoclonus		+	
Ataxia	±	+	
Seizures		+	+
Vomiting			+
Cortical blindness			+
Hemiparesis			+

Table 12. Symptoms of mitochondrial disorders. See text for abbreviations.

MOVEMENT DISORDERS AND ATAXIA

A. **See also:** Pediatric Movement Disorders, p. 114.

B. **Terminology:** "Movement disorders" tends to include only problems with a presumed basal ganglia cause. "Extrapyramidal symptoms" is an old-fashioned term, used in distinction to pyramidal sx from corticospinal lesions.

C. **Movement disorder consult service jingle:** "Trouble with tone? Just get on the phone. Jerky or stiff? We're there in a jiff."

D. **H&P:** What tasks are difficult? Nature and frequency of falls. Associated depression, dementia, incontinence. Alcohol, benzodiazepine, or neuroleptic use. Assess facial expression, saccades, voice, handwriting, involuntary movements, speed, amplitude, tone, ability to rise from a chair, posture, postural reflexes, gait base, arm swing, festination, freezing, turning Romberg sign, weakness, ataxia.

E. **Gait disorders:**
   1. **Types of gait disorders:**
      a. **Spastic gait:** Stiff, circumducted leg, arm often flexed. From corticospinal lesion.
      b. **Ataxic gait:** Lurching, wide-based, but rarely falls. From cerebellar system lesion.
      c. **Akinetic-rigid gait:** Stooped, shuffling, trouble starting and stopping, often with tremor, decreased arm swing, poor postural reflexes. From basal ganglia lesion.
      d. **Frontal gait:** Gait apraxia—trouble lifting feet, retropulsion, although leg movements may be normal in bed. Often mild ataxia. From cortical or white matter lesions; normal pressure hydrocephalus (see p. 34).
      e. **Neuropathic gait:** High-stepping (steppage gait), feet slap, Romberg positive, distal weakness. From peripheral nerve lesion.
      f. **Spastic-ataxic gait:** A characteristic bouncing gait. Often seen in multiple sclerosis, Chiari malformation, hydrocephalus in young people.
      g. **Others:** Dystonic gait, choreic gait, action myoclonus, leg action tremor, frontal gait, abasia-astasia (psychogenic).

F. **Cerebellar/brainstem movement disorders:** Ataxia, dysmetria; often with vertigo, nystagmus, N/V, irregular prosody.
   1. **Acute:** Bleed, infarct, toxins, drugs. Secondary edema may be lifethreatening and require rapid neurosurgical intervention
   2. **Subacute:** Tumor, postinfectious cerebellitis, vasculitis, toxins, drugs.
   3. **Chronic progressive:** Alcoholism, Wilson's dz, drugs, toxins, Creutzfeldt-Jakob dz, hereditary cerebellar degeneration, hereditary metabolic dz, paraneoplastic syndromes.
   4. **DDx:** Other gait disorders, above.

G. **Basal ganglia movement disorders:**
   1. **Circuitry:** Lesions that affect the excitatory pathway through the internal pallidum cause hypokinetic movement disorders, those that affect the inhibitory pathway through the external pallidum cause hyperkinetic ones.
   2. **Akathisia:** Motor restlessness. Often transient side effect of neuroleptic. Try propranolol 10-20 mg tid, clonidine 0.1 mg bid, or clonazepam 0.5-1.0 mg bid.
   3. **Asterixis:** Irregular, slow, tremor-like flapping of hands, trunk, caused by temporary lapses of tone.

       a. Causes: Usually metabolic, e.g. liver failure.

       b. Rx: Treat underlying cause.

4. Choreoathetosis: Chorea is involuntary, rapid movements, often incorporated into voluntary movements. Athetosis is slower, more writhing.

    a. Causes of choreoathetosis:

      1) **Chemicals:** Especially neuroleptics.

      2) **Immune-mediated:** Sydenham's chorea, lupus, chorea gravidorum,....

      3) **Hereditary disorders:** Huntington's, Wilson's, Hallervorden-Spatz dz, idiopathic torsion dystonia,....

         a) **Huntington's dz:** Autosomal dominant CAG sequence repeat, genetic test available. Presents usually in adulthood with chorea or psychiatric sx.

    b. Rx of choreoathetosis: Neuroleptics e.g. haloperidol—start 0.5 mg tid, up to 8-16 mg qd.

5. Dyskinesia: A general term for abnormal involuntary movements. Often a side effect of drugs for Parkinson's dz.

6. Dystonia: Involuntary maintenance of abnormal posture, expression, or limb position. Often task-dependent and relieved by sensory tricks.

    a. DDx of dystonia: Spasticity, musculoskeletal lesion,....

    b. Causes of dystonia:

      1) **Acute:** Reaction to antiemetic or neuroleptic, carbon monoxide, stroke,....

      2) **Chronic:**

         a) **Focal:** Torticollis, blepharospasm, writer's cramp, Meige's syndrome (lip smacking and blepharospasm), spasmodic dysphonia,....

         b) **Global, hereditary:** See pediatric dystonia, p. 115, and causes of choreoathetosis, above.

    c. Rx of dystonia:

      1) **Acute dystonic reaction to a neuroleptic:** Diphenhydramine 50 mg IV/IM.

      2) **Chronic dystonia:**

         a) **Anticholinergics:** e.g. trihexyphenidyl. Start 1 mg qd, to 20-50 tid or more.

         b) **Botulinum toxin injections:** For focal dystonia. Effect lasts 3-4 mo.

         c) **Other:** Sinemet, baclofen, diazepam.

7. Myoclonus: Brief, monophasic, irregular jerks in different body parts. Often triggered by sensory stimuli.

    a. DDx: Clonus, tremor, chorea, focal seizure, myoclonic epilepsy.

    b. Causes of myoclonus: Metabolic or hypoxic encephalopathy, seizure, benign essential myoclonus (including nocturnal myoclonus), physiological myoclonus (sleep jerks), drugs (e.g. opiates),....

    c. Rx of myoclonus

      1) **Clonazepam** (benzodiazepine): Start 0.5 mg tid, to 2 tid

      2) **Valproic acid:** Start 15 mg/kg qd divided bid-tid.

3) **5-OH-tryptophan:** Start 100 mg bid, increase by 100 bid q 3 days to total of 500-750 bid. Can give carbidopa to decrease extracerebral metabolism.

8. Parkinsonism:

a. **Pathophysiology:** Dopaminergic neurons in the substantia nigra pars compacta die, causing dopamine depletion in the striatum (caudate nucleus and putamen).

b. **H&P:** Asymmetric rest tremor (see p. 62), bradykinesia, cogwheel rigidity. Masked face, decreased arm swing, postural instability, festination. Response to Sinemet; on/off phenomena, depression. Later, cognitive changes, hallucinations on drugs, orthostasis, and bladder changes.

c. **Tests:** None, unless there are atypical features.

d. **DDx of idiopathic Parkinson's dz** (PD):

1) **"Parkinson's plus" syndromes:** Usually poor response to Sinemet. They include progressive supranuclear palsy (more falling and gaze palsy); Lewy body dz (early hallucinations and delir-

| Age < 50 |
| Sudden onset or fast progression |
| Early falls |
| Early dementia |
| Unusual tremor or myoclonus |
| Early autonomic disturbances |
| Poor levodopa response |
| Gaze palsies |
| Marked dysarthria or dysphagia |
| Family history |

Table 13. Symptoms not typical of PD.

ium); and multiple system atrophy including Shy-Drager syndrome (more autonomic dysfunction), striatonigral degeneration (spasticity, no tremor), and olivopontocerebellar atrophy (ataxia; pseudobulbar signs),....

2) **Chemicals:** e.g. neuroleptics (including antiemetics), manganese, carbon monoxide,....

3) **Other:** Essential tremor, depression, arthritis, focal basal ganglia lesions, spasticity, NPH, repeated head trauma (dementia pugilistica), postencephalitic, Creutzfeldt-Jacob dz,....

e. **Rx of PD:** See p.135 for dopaminergic drugs and doses.

1) **Early dz:** Selegiline is sometimes used first.

2) **Well-established:** Levodopa + carbidopa (Sinemet).

3) **Severe, on-off symptoms or dopa dyskinesias:**
   a) **Change Sinemet frequency or dose.**
   b) **Add a dopamine agonist and lower Sinemet:** See agonists.
   c) **Surgery:** Pallidotomy, pallidal or subthalamic stimulator.

4) **Levodopa-resistant PD tremor:** Anticholinergics sometimes help. See Dystonia, above.

5) **Hallucinations or agitation:** Atypical neuroleptics, e.g. quetiapine 25 mg qhs or clozapine 25 mg. Avoid haloperidol.

6) **Autonomic insufficiency:** Consider vascular stockings, high-salt diet, head of bed up 10 degrees (at home, place bricks under bed), fludrocortisone 0.1 mg qd, or midodrine 10 mg tid.

7) **Symptom worsening during an acute illness:** Increasing meds usually doesn't help and may increase confusion.

9. Neuroleptic-induced movement disorders: See p. 136.

10.Serotonin-induced movement disorders: See Serotonin syndrome, p. 130.

11.Tics: Quick, repetitive, coordinated movements or vocalizations, driven by urge, partly repressible.

    a. DDx: Tourette's syndrome, Sydenham's chorea, Wilson's dz, Lesch-Nyhan's syndrome, myoclonus,....

    b. Rx: (Generally not well-tolerated)

        1) **Clonidine** (central α–agonist): Start 0.1 mg bid, to 2 mg qd.

        2) **Pimozide** (or other D_2 antagonist): Start 1-2 mg qd, to 8-16 mg qd.

12.Tremor: Oscillation from alternating contraction of antagonist muscles.

    a. DDx: Focal seizure, segmental myoclonus, chorea.

    b. Rest (parkinsonian) tremor: 3-5 Hz, decreases during movement, often asymmetric, "pill-rolling."

    c. Action tremors: Worse with movement.

        1) **Physiologic tremor:** Normal, low-amplitude, 8-13 Hz. Worse with adrenergic stimulation (anxiety, caffeine, hyperthyroidism, sedative withdrawal,...).

        2) **Essential (benign) tremor:** Usually hereditary, 4-8 Hz. Rx includes

            a) **Propranolol:** Start 10-20 mg tid, to 60-200 mg qd.

            b) **Primidone:** Start 50 mg qd, to 125 tid.

            c) **Surgery:** Thalamotomy; stimulator implant.

        3) **Cerebellar tremor:** Strictly, dysmetria. Oscillations worsen as limb approaches target.

        4) **Rubral tremor:** Midbrain tremor would be a better term. Violent beating or flapping. An example is hemiballism from a subthalamic nucleus lesion.

NEUROMUSCULAR DISORDERS

A. See also: Peripheral neuropathy, p. 72, Weakness, p. 99.

B. Presenting clinical features:

	Anterior horn cell	Neuropathic	Neuromuscular junction	Myopathic
Distrib. of weakness	Asymmetric	Symmetric distal	Eyes, face, proximal	Symmetrical limb > face
Atrophy	Marked, early	Moderate	None	Slight early, marked late
Sensory loss	None	Yes	None	None
Classic features	Fasciculations, cramps, tremor	Sensory and motor	Diurnal fluctuation	Weak; sometimes pain
Reflexes	Increased or decreased	Lost early	Normal	Decr. if weakness severe

Table 14. Presenting features of neuromuscular diseases.

C. Abnormal muscle activity:

    1. Clonus: Repetitive unidirectional contraction of a muscle group.

2. **Fasciculations:** Random twitching of a muscle fiber group.
3. **Fibrillations:** Random single fiber twitching.
4. **Myotonia:** Delayed muscle relaxation, often triggered by percussion. Worse in cold, improves with exercise
5. **Myokymia:** Repetitive, undulating fasciculations.

D. **Pulmonary function in neuromuscular dz:** Characterized by decreased vital capacity (VC), hypercarbia. A bedside test of VC is to have the pt. count aloud while maximally exhaling—normal > 40. Consider intubating if < 20, or for VC < 18 mg/kg. Oxygen saturation monitors are not adequate tests, as desaturation may only occur late. For pulmonary function test findings, see p. 185.

E. **Amyotrophic lateral sclerosis**
   1. **H&P:** Weakness without cognitive, sensory, or ANS dysfunction. Combination of upper and lower motor neuron signs. Frequently hand atrophy, foot drop, leg spasticity, bulbar sx, fasciculations, cramps. Family history?
   2. **DDx:** CIDP, other motor system atrophies, cervical spinal cord injury, MS, myasthenia, paraneoplastic syndrome, multifocal motor neuropathy with conduction block, heavy metal poisoning, HIV, diabetic amyotrophy, post-polio syndrome,....
   3. **Tests:**
      a. **Consider peripheral neuropathy workup:** See p. 72.
      b. **EMG:** Much denervation and reinnervation (fasciculations, fibrillations, polyphasic increase in amplitude of motor units, normal conduction speed).
      c. **Biopsy:** Usually not indicated. Shows neurogenic atrophy.
   4. **Rx:**
      a. **Riluzole:** (Rilutek) 50 mg PO bid. Slightly slows progression.
      b. **Supportive:** e.g. splints, G-tube, mechanical ventilation.

F. **Botulism:** Preformed toxin blocks acetylcholine release from neuromuscular junction, causing bradycardia, ophthalmoplegia, and bulbar, respiratory, and somatic paralysis with intact mentation and sensation. For EMG findings, see p. 33. Treat with antitoxin.

G. **Lambert-Eaton myasthenic syndrome:** Blockage of presynaptic acetylcholine release, probably from antibodies to a voltage-gated calcium channel. 50% of pts. have an underlying cancer.
   1. **H&P:** Unlike myasthenia, often begins with proximal limb rather than cranial nerve weakness, and excercise may transiently improve rather than worsen weakness.
   2. **Tests:** Similar to myasthenia, below, plus workup for occult cancer.
   3. **Rx:** Treat underlying cancer. 3,4-Diaminopyridine (DAP) 5-25 mg PO tid or qid. Pyridostigmine is not as effective as it is in myasthenia. Avoid drugs that affect the neuromuscular junction (see p. 65).

H. **Myasthenia gravis:** Caused by antibodies to the acetylcholine receptor (measurable in 75% of pts.). 10% of pts. have a thymoma.
   1. **H&P:** Sx worse at end of day or after repeated use? Diplopia? Trouble swallowing? Shortness of breath? Recent infection or med change? Check vital capacity (see hypoventilation in neuromuscular dz, p. 63), sustained eye elevation, neck strength, repeated standing. Ice pack on eyelid may improve myasthenic ptosis. Should have nor-

mal pupils, sensory, and reflex exam. Reflexes may be depressed if limbs are very weak.
2. **DDx:** Guillain-Barré syndrome, CIDP, botulism, motor neuron dz, organophosphate poisoning, myopathy, muscular dystrophy, thyroid dz.
3. **Tests:** Edrophonium test (if pt. currently symptomatic), acetylcholine receptor Ab, EMG with 3-Hz repetitive stimulation and single fiber studies (see p. 33), chest CT for thymoma, electrolytes, Ca/phos/Mg, CPK, ANA, RF, TSH, antithyroid Ab.
    a. **Edrophonium test (Tensilon test):** A short-acting cholinesterase inhibitor. 1-2 mg IV. If no change, give additional 8 mg (i.e. total 10 mg). Need double-blind, placebo control. Do not perform if pupils miotic (suggests cholinergic crisis). Perform with a cardiac monitor if the pt. is elderly. Have atropine ready for bradycardia.
4. **Myasthenic crisis and cholinergic crisis:** Both present with weakness. <u>Both are emergencies</u>, because of the danger of respiratory collapse. May have both at once.

	Myasthenic crisis	Cholinergic crisis
Heart rate	Tachycardic	Bradycardic
Muscles	Flaccid	Flaccid, + fasciculations
Pupil	Normal or large	Small
Skin	Pale, sometimes cool	Red, warm
Secretions	No change	Increased
Edrophonium test	Improves strength	Increases weakness

Table 15. Distinguishing myasthenic and cholinergic crises.

   a. **Tests:** Bedside vital capacity, cardiac monitor.
   b. **Rx of myasthenic crisis:**
      1) **Cholinergics:** Prostigmine 0.5 mg IV push, then pyridostigmine 24 mg in 500 ml D5 1/2 NS.
      2) **Respiratory support:** Admit to ICU, follow vital capacity, intubate if VC is < 15-18 ml/kg, or if aspiration risk. Remember that O_2 saturation is not sensitive; pt. will become hypercarbic before becoming hypoxic.
      3) **Remove precipitants:** Drugs, infection, heat.
      4) **Plasmapheresis:** ~6x in 2 wk.
      5) **Steroids:** Consider 60 mg methylprednisolone IV qd. Steroids may acutely worsen weakness; monitor closely.
   c. **Rx of cholinergic crisis:** Similar to myasthenic crisis, since pyridostigmine overdose is usually a response to worsening myasthenia.
      1) **Atropine:** 2 mg IV for nonmuscle effects.
      2) **Ipratroprium inhaler:** For bronchospasm.
5. **Outpatient rx of myasthenia:**
   a. **Pyridostigmine (Mestinon):** Start 30-60 mg q4-6h. Side effects: diarrhea, urinary frequency, bradycardia, cholinergic crisis.
   b. **Prednisone:** Pt. may worsen for first few weeks. Start 10 mg qd as outpatient, or admit for more agressive load. Increase slowly.
   c. **Azathioprine:** Start 50 mg q am; increase to 150 mg q am over 3 wk. Takes months to affect symptoms. Monitor LFTs/CBC weekly

x 2 mo, then monthly.
    d. **Thymectomy:** In young pts., or if thymoma. Works better if done early.
  6. **Drugs to avoid in myasthenia and Eaton-Lambert syndrome:**
    a. **Anticholinergics.**
    b. **Cardiovascular:** β-block, antiarrythmics (these can sometimes cause transient drug-induced myasthenia).
    c. **Antibiotic:** Gentamycin, tetracycline, clindamycin (penicillin and erythromycin are better).
    d. **Neurological:** Phenytoin, lithium, neuroleptics, muscle relaxants,...
    e. **Antimalarial:** Chloroquine.
I. **Myositis and myopathy**
  1. **H&P:** Swallowing, diplopia, family history. Myotonia (can't release grip), symmetry of weakness, edema, proximal vs. distal, rash (violet lids, subungual telangiectasias). Bowel, bladder should be normal.
  2. **Causes:** Poly- or. dermatomyositis (often secondary to malignancy), thyroid, alcohol, steroids,....
  3. **DDx:** Muscular dystrophy, myasthenia, MS, metabolic, infection (HIV, syphilis, parasites), lupus, sarcoid, cord lesion, ischemia, polymyalgia rheumatica, diabetic amyotrophy, Behçet's syndrome, rhabdomyolysis, glycogen storage dz,....
  4. **Tests:** CPK, EMG, ESR, ANA, TSH, MCV, muscle biopsy.
  5. **Rx:**
    a. **Steroids:** Prednisone 60-100 mg qd until improvement, then 40 qd x several months. If patient is already on steroids, try tapering them – it may be steroid myopathy.
    b. **Immunosuppression:** Follow WBC, LFTs qwk, then qmo.
      1) **Aazthioprine:** Effects take months. Start 50 qd x 1 wek, then 100 qd x 1 wk, then 150 qd.
      2) **Methotrexate:** 0.4 mg/kg/treatment IV at first treatment, increasing to 0.8 mg/kg in 3 wk. Dose weekly at first, then every 2-3 wk.

NEUROSURGICAL PROCEDURES

A. **See also:** Intracranial hemorrhage, p. 50; Intracranial pressure, p. 53; Spinal cord, p. 85; Trauma, p. 89; Brain tumors, p. 90; Spine tumors, p. 94; Pediatric tumors, p. 120; Pediatric head circumference abnormalities, p. 107.
B. **Generic pre-op orders:**
  1. **NPO except meds after midnight:** IV fluids if scheduled as second case.
  2. **Compression boots on call to OR.**
  3. **Void on call to OR.**
  4. **Pre-op meds:** Consider
    a. **Steroids:** e.g. dexamethasone 10 mg PO at night, 10 mg IV on call, or stress doses for those on chronic steroids.
    b. **Prophylactic Abx:** e.g. 1 g cefazolin or vancomycin on call.
    c. **Ranitidine:** e.g. 150 mg PO at night, 50 mg IV on call.

      d. Anticonvulsants.

      e. Sleeping pill.

C. Pre-op check: Write a pre-op note in the chart documenting

    1. Vital signs and neurological exam.

    2. Labs: Electrolytes, BUN, Cr, CBC, platelets, PT, PTT, anticonvulsant levels, UA, EKG, CXR.

    3. Blood: Type and hold 2 U (4 for vascular cases).

    4. Consent.

    5. Plan.

D. Post-op orders:

    1. Admit: To postanesthesia care unit, transfer to ICU when stable.

    2. Vital signs: q15min x 4h, then q1h; temperature q4h x 3d, then q8h; craniotomy checks.

    3. Activity: Bedrest, HOB elevated 20-30° for craniotomies. Compression boots or hose. Incentive spirometry q2h while awake (except if post-transsphenoidal).

    4. Diet: NPO except meds.

    5. I/Os: q1h. If no indwelling catheter, straight catheter q6h PRN.

    6. IV fluids: e.g. NS + 20 mEq KCl/L at 75 ml/h.

    7. O$_2$: e.g. 2 L per nasal cannula.

    8. Meds: Consider

      a. Steroids: e.g. dexamethasone 4 mg IV q6h, or stress doses for those on chronic steroids.

      b. Ranitidine: 50 mg IV q8h.

      c. Anticonvulsants.

      d. Nitroprusside: To keep SBP < 160.

      e. Codeine: 30-60 mg PO/IM q 3h prn HA.

      f. Acetaminophen: 650 mg PO/PR q4h prn temp. > 100.5 F.

E. Post-op check:

    1. Events.

    2. Vital signs, I/Os.

    3. General exam, wound check.

    4. Neurological exam.

    5. Labs.

    6. Plan.

F. Post-op deterioration: Usually requires emergent CT.

    1. DDx: Hemorrhage, infarction, seizure, tension pneumocephalus, infection, cardiac or pulmonary event, persistent anesthetic effect (unlikely in a patient who was initially doing well post-op.)

    2. Seizures: Intubate pts. who do not rapidly regain consciousness, or have labored breathing. Draw anticonvulsant levels and bolus with additional anticonvulsants —do not wait for levels.

G. Craniotomy:

    1. Frontal, temporal, parietal and occipital craniotomies: For access to cortical and subcortical lesions; also for access to the ventricles. Transcallosal approaches have increased risk of venous infarction; usually require preoperative angiography.

    2. Posterior fossa (suboccipital) craniotomy: Used to reach the cerebellopontine angle, one vertebral artery, or as an extreme lateral approach to the anterolateral brainstem. In addition to the routine post-op issues described above, •

    a. **Closely monitor respirations:** Pts. may benefit from 24-48 h post-op intubation, since posterior fossa complications often have respiratory arrest as the presenting sign.

    b. **Keep SBP < 160:** with nitroprusside if necessary. Sudden changes in BP may indicate a posterior fossa hematoma or edema.

    c. **Posterior fossa hematoma or edema:** Presents with sudden changes in breathing or BP; pupils, consciousness, and ICP are not affected until late. Rx is rapid intubation, ventricular drainage (through prophylactically placed burr hole, if possible), and immediate reoperation. A CT scan may dangerously delay treatment.

    d. **Watch for CSF leak through wound or nose.** This is often a sign of CSF obstruction, and the leak may not resolve until you shunt the CSF. When you see a leak, elevate the HOB, and reinforce the incision with more sutures or several coats of colloidon.

    e. **If corneal reflex is poor,** due to 5th or 7th nerve injury, protect eye with drops, ointment, or patch.

  3. **Pterional craniotomy:** To reach anterior circulation and basilar tip aneurysms, cavernous sinus, and suprasellar tumors. The craniotomy is centered over the depression of the sphenoid ridge. When the sella is accessed, consider post-op complications of transsphenoidal surgery, below.

H. Transsphenoidal surgery: Used for sellar tumors without significant suprasellar extension.

  1. **Post-op complications:** Diabetes insipidus (see p.162), adrenal insufficiency, hypothyroidism, hypogonadism, secondary empty sella syndrome (visual loss from chiasm retracting into sella), infection, CSF rhinorrhea, carotid artery rupture, nasal septal perforation.

  2. **Post-op orders:**

    a. **I/Os q1h,** with urine specific gravity q4h, and electrolytes with osmolarity q6h.

    b. **IV fluids:** D5 1/2 NS + 20 mEq KCl/L at 75-100 ml/h, plus replace urine output ml for ml with 1/2 NS.

    c. **Abx:** Continue pre-op regimen until nasal packs removed.

    d. **Steroid taper:** e.g., hydrocortisone 50 mg IM/IV/PO bid, taper 10 mg/dose qd. Test am cortisol 24 h after stopping steroids.

    e. **Activity:** No incentive spirometry or drinking through a straw, to avoid aspirating the sinus fat graft.

I. CSF access and decompression techniques: All increase risk of CNS infection.

  1. **Ventriculostomy:** AKA intraventricular catheter or external ventricular drainage. For temporary ICP monitoring and CSF drainage. May be inserted at the bedside. Usually done in non-dominant hemisphere.

    a. **Orders:** Hang bag 15 cm above head; drain for pressure > 15 cm. Empiric nafcillin 2 g IV q4h.

    b. **Weaning:** Can sometimes wean even if output high (~150 ml qd). Clamp; open if pressure greater than 20; then leave open until it decreases to 15.

  2. **Ventricular shunts:** Usually ventriculoperitoneal; occasionally ven-

triculo-atrial, ventriculo-pleural, or lumbo-peritoneal. For permanent CSF drainage. Inserted in OR.

   a. Hardware: May contain valves to prevent overshunting, reservoirs to allow CSF taps, or tumor filters to prevent seeding.
   b. Complications: Infection, undershunting or occlusion, overshunting (can cause headache or SDH).

3. Shunt or reservoir tap: To access the reservoir, shave scalp, iodine prep for 5 min, and insert a 25-gauge butterfly needle at an oblique angle.

4. Ommaya reservoir: An indwelling reservoir attached to a ventricular catheter. It allows intrathecal chemotherapy or Abx, or recurrent CSF aspiration.

5. Lumbar drain: Temporary catheter placed to lower CSF pressure, usually to treat postoperative CSF leak. Pt. should be on Abx while drain is in place.

PAIN

A. H&P: Location, quality, duration, intensity, aggravating and relieving factors, h/o trauma, disability, litigation, drugs tried, other treatments, imaging work, psychiatric history, strength, range of motion, straight leg raise, pin prick and light touch sensation, skin color and temperature, dystrophic skin changes.

B. Pain treatment by cause:
   1. Bone pain: NSAIDS (especially aspirin) + acetaminophen, steroids, opiates. XRT or strontium-90 for metastases. A corset may help compression fractures.
   2. Compression or nerve ischemia: Selective death of large fibers causes disinhibited small fibers, thus paresthesias.
   3. Gout: NSAIDS or colchicine; allopurinol (not in acute flare), keep pt. hydrated; avoid loop diuretics.
   4. Liver or other organ metastases: Steroids.
   5. Mouth pain from ulceration: Diphenhydramine, xylocaine, and kaopectate liquids in 1:1:1 ratio; give 15 ml q3h prn.
   6. Neuropathic pain:
      a. Drugs: TCAs or anticonvulsants.
      b. Surgery: Nerve decompression may help if movement exacerbates paresthesias.
      c. Treat accompanying depression.
   7. Complex regional pain syndrome (includes sympathetically mediated pain or reflex sympathetic dystrophy): Look for altered color or temperature of skin, burning pain, skin hypersensitivity to light touch, trophic changes, stiff joints.
      a. Topical lidocaine: May help skin hypersensitivity.
      b. IV phentolamine test: Can help predict the effect of sympathetic nerve block. Check EKG first.
      c. Sympathetic nerve block: May help if signs of sympathetically mediated pain (e.g. skin cold, damp).
   8. Trigeminal neuralgia: Lancinating, often with trigger points. Often associated with MS. Rarely from dental dz or brain tumor. Try carba-

mazepine 100-400 tid, gabapentin, phenytoin, baclofen, or lamictal.
Consider surgery.
9. **Zoster (shingles):**
   a. **Acute:** If pt. over 50 or lesions last > 72 h, give antiherpetic, e.g.
      famcyclovir. Try lidocaine cream.
   b. **Postherpetic pain:**
      1) **Early nerve blocks.**
      2) **Constant pain:** Try a TCA.
      3) **Lancinating:** Try gabapentin or other anticonvulsant.

PARANEOPLASTIC SYNDROMES

A. **Incidence:** Although rare (1% of cancer patients), paraneoplastic syndrome precede the diagnosis of cancer in about 60% of those cases.

Syndrome	Clinical features	Antibody	Common cancer
BRAIN			
Brainstem encephalitis	Ataxia, cranial n. or motor dysfunction, abnormal CSF	Hu	Small cell lung cancer (SCLC)
Limbic encephalopathy	Depression, confusion, abnormal CSF	Hu	SCLC
Subacute cerebellar degeneration	Ataxia, dysarthria, nystagmus, nl CSF	Yo; Purkinje cell	Breast, ovary; SCLC, Hodgkins
Opsoclonus, myoclonus	Jerky eye and limb movement	Ri	Lung, breast
Isolated CNS angiitis			Hodgkin's dz
Retinal degeneration	Loss of vision	Retinal	SCLC
SPINAL CORD			
Subacute necrotizing myelopathy	Weakness, sensory loss	IgG	SCLC
Motor neuron dz	Weakness, fasciculations		Lymphomas
Stiff man syndrome	Painful spasms	IgG	Lung, lymphoma, breast, thymoma
PERIPHERAL NERVE			
Subacute sensory neuropathy	Dysesthesias	Neuronal IgG	SCLC
Gammopathy-associated neuropathy	Sensory loss, weakness, areflexia	Monoclonal Ig	Myeloma
Guillain-Barré (AIDP)	Rapid weakness, areflexia	IgG	Lymphoma
NEUROMUSCULAR JUNCTION			
Lambert-Eaton syndrome	Proximal weakness, areflexia, eyes spared	Calcium channel	SCLC
Myasthenia gravis	Weakness, areflexia, eyes often involved	Acetylcholine receptor	Thymoma
MUSCLE			
Dermato- or polymyositis	Weakness, high CPK	Muscle	Breast, lung, GI, uterine, ovarian

Table 16. Paraneoplastic syndromes.

PERIPHERAL NERVES

A. **See also:** Peripheral neuropathy, p. 72.
B. **Spinal level by disc:** See Table 1, Figure 2.
C. **Spinal level by function:**
   1. **Movement:**
      a. **Neck:** C1-C4.

    b. Diaphragm: C3-C5

    c. Shoulder: Abduction and lateral rotation is C5. Adduction and medial rotation is C6-C8.

    d. Elbow: Flexion is C5-C6. Extension is C6-C8.

    e. Wrist: C6-8. Extension is radial nerve. Flexion is median and ulnar nerve.

    f. Hand: Finger abduction and adduction are ulnar nerve (C8-T1). Grip is median nerve. Finger extension is radial nerve.

    g. Thumb test: Can separate radial, median, and ulnar nerve lesions by thumb movements. Mnemonic is <u>RUM</u>: <u>R</u>adial extends, <u>U</u>lnar adducts, and <u>M</u>edian abducts. Flexion and extension are in the plane of the palm; abduction and adduction are at right angles to the palm.

    h. Intercostals: T2-T9.

    i. Abdominals: Upper is T9-T10. Lower is T11-T12.

    j. Hip: Flexion is L2-L4, adduction is L3-L4, abduction is L5-S1.

    k. Knee: Extension is L2-L4; flexion is L4-S1.

    l. Foot: Dorsiflexion is L4-S1; plantar flexion is S1-S2.

    m. Bladder, anal sphincter: S2-S4.

  2. Sensation:

    a. Arm: Shoulders: C4; inner forearm: C6; outer forearm: T1; thumb: C6; fifth finger: C8.

    b. Leg: Front of thigh: L2; medial calf: L4; lateral calf: L5; fifth toe: S1; midline buttocks: S3.

D. Spinal level by nerve

  1. See: Peripheral neuropathy, p. 72, for sx of common trauma and entrapment syndromes.

  2. Arm:

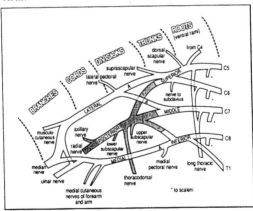

Figure 8. The brachial plexus. (From Warwick R, and Williams P. *Gray's Anatomy*, 35th ed. Edinburgh: Churchill Livingstone, 1973, with permission.)

    a. Brachial plexus: C5-T1.

      1) **Plexi:**

a) **Upper plexus:** C5-C6. Deltoids, biceps, supra- and infra-spinatus.
b) **Middle plexus:** C7.
c) **Lower plexus:** C8-T1.

2) **Cords:** Upper-mid-lower plexi recombine to form three cords: Lateral and medial cord then recombine to form median nerve.

a) **Lateral cord** (from upper + middle plexus) forms musculo-cutaneous nerve, lateral anterior thoracic nerve, median nerve.
b) **Posterior cord** (from upper, middle, and lower plexus) forms radial nerve, axillary nerve, and subscapular nerve.
c) **Medial cord** (from lower plexus) forms ulnar nerve, medial cutaneous nerve, median nerve.

b. **Nerves of arm:** Note that any weakness of both flexors and extensors, or of all intrinsic hand muscles, implies that the lesion cannot be a mononeuropathy.

1) **Long thoracic nerve:** C5-C7. Serratus anterior. Test: scapula wings when pt. presses arm forward against a wall..
2) **Axillary nerve:** C5-C6. Deltoid, etc. Test: abduct arm > 90 degrees.
3) **Musculocutaneous nerve:** C5-C6. Biceps.
4) **Radial nerve:** C5-C8, es. C7. Extensors (triceps, wrist and finger), supinator, brachioradialis.
5) **Median nerve:** C6-T1. Flexors except ulnar: most forearm flexors, flex. dig. superior; all pronators. Hand: LOAF muscles (Lumbricals 1 and 2, Opp. pollicis., Abd. poll. brev., Flex. poll. brev.)
6) **Ulnar nerve:** C8-T1. Flexor digitorum profundus 3 and 4, flexor carpi ulnaris. Most of intrinsic hand (except LOAF muscles above): thumb adductors and flexors, interossei, lumbricals 3 and 4, hypothenar muscles.

3. **Leg:**
   a. **Femoral nerve:** L2-4.
      1) **Function:** Extend knee.
      2) **Muscles:** Iliopsoas, quadriceps, sartorius, rectus femoris.
   b. **Obturator nerve:** L2-4.
      1) **Function:** Adduct leg.
      2) **Muscles:** Adductor longus, brevis, and magnus; gracilus, pectineus,....
   c. **Sciatic nerve** (tibial and peroneal nerve): L4-S2.
      1) **Function:** Extends/abducts hip, flex knee, all foot movements.
         a) **Deep peroneal nerve:** Extends toes and ankle.
         b) **Superficial peroneal nerve:** Everts foot.
         c) **Tibial nerve:** Superficial tibial flexes foot; deep tibial flexes toes.
      2) **Muscles:** Semitendinosus and -membranosus, biceps femoris, gastrocnemius, soleus, foot muscles,....

E. **Spinal level by reflex:**
   1. **Cervical:** Biceps is C5-C6. Supinator is C5-C6. Triceps is C6-C8.
   2. **Thoracic:** Scratch toward navel. Contraction with scratching above

navel is T8-T10; below navel is T10-T12.
3. **Lumbar:** Knee is L2-L4. Ankle is S1-S2. Babinski is L4-S2.

PERIPHERAL NEUROPATHY

A. **See also:** Peripheral nerves, p. 69, weakness, p. 99.
B. **H&P:** Weakness, numbness, pain, distal vs. proximal, autonomic sx (GI motility, BP, temperature regulation), bowel and bladder function, injuries or deformities, alcoholism, diabetes, medications, HIV status, reflexes.
C. **DDx:** CNS lesion; myopathy, metabolic (e.g. paresthesias from alkalosis),....
D. **Tests:** Consider EMG/NCS, KCl/Ca/Mg/Phos, CPK, B_{12}, MCV, ESR, TSH, hemoglobin A1c, Lyme titer, HIV, ANA.
E. **Types of neuropathy:**
  1. **Polyneuropathy:** Usually axonal degeneration or demyelination.
  2. **Mononeuropathy or mononeuropathy multiplex:** Usually entrapment, trauma, or process that disrupts the vasa nervosum.
  3. **Sensorimotor.**
  4. **Motor.**
  5. **Sensory.**
F. **Causes of neuropathy:**
  1. **A mnemonic for causes:** DANG THERAPIST: DM, Alcohol, Nutritional, GBS, Trauma, Hereditary, Endocrine/Entrapment, Renal/Radiation, AIDS/Amyloid, Paraprotein/Porphyria, Infectious (e.g. leprosy), Systemic/Sarcoid, Toxins.
  2. **Causes categorized:** By time course, distribution, and EMG finding:
    a. **Acute, generalized:**
      1) **Axonal degeneration:**
        a) **Infections:** Lyme, HIV, EBV, hepatitis, CMV.
        b) **Miscellaneous:** porphyria, axonal Guillain-Barré syndrome, ICU neuropathy.
      2) **Demyelination:** Guillain-Barré syndrome, arsenic, infections, e.g. HIV and diphtheria.
    b. **Chronic, generalized:**
      1) **Axonal degeneration:**
        a) **Nutritional:** Alcohol, folate, vitamins B_6, B_{12}, or E.
        b) **Toxic:** Phenytoin, vincristine, heavy metals, acrylamide, etc.
        c) **Endocrine:** DM, hypothyroidism.
        d) **Infectious:** HIV, Lyme.
        e) **Genetic:** Charcot-Marie-Tooth (CMT) type II, familial amyloidosis, Friedreich's ataxia, etc.
        f) **Lipid problems:** Fabry's dz, Tangier dz, Bassen-Kornzweig dz.
        g) **Other:** Uremia, vasculitis.
      2) **Demyelination:**
        a) **Uniform slowing on EMG:** CMT types 1A, 1B, and X; myelin dysmetabolism, e.g. metachromatic leukodystrophy, Refsum dz, Krabbe dz.

  b) **Nonuniform slowing:**
- **Infectious or inflammatory:** HIV, CIDP, multifocal neuropathy with conduction block.
- **Paraprotein:** Lymphoma, myeloma, POEMS syndrome (<u>p</u>olyneuropathy with <u>o</u>rganomegaly, <u>e</u>ndocrinopathy, <u>m</u>-protein, and <u>s</u>kin changes), Waldenström's macroglobulinemia, MGUS (<u>m</u>onoclonal gammopathy of <u>u</u>ncertain <u>s</u>ignificance), cryoglobulinemia.

 c. Mononeuropathy multiplex: (multifocal or asymmetric)
  1) **Axonal:**
   a) **Vascular:** DM, vasculitis (polyarteritis nodosa, Wegener's, giant cell arteritis, hypersensitivity), connective tissue dz, subacute bacterial endocarditis.
   b) **Infectious or inflammatory:** HIV, Lyme, leprosy, VZV, hepatitis A, sarcoid.
   c) **Neoplastic:** Neurofibromatosis, leukemia, direct local invasion.
   d) **Miscellaneous:** Genetic ,e.g. inherited brachial plexus neuropathy; traumatic, e.g. multiple compressions.
  2) **Demyelinating:**
   a) **Inflammatory:** Guillain-Barré; multifocal motor neuropathy with conduction block.
   b) **Genetic:** Hereditary neuropathy with liability to pressure palsies (HNPP).
   c) **Multiple compressions.**

G. Specific neuropathies:
 1. Inflammatory demyelinating polyneuropathies: e.g. Guillain-Barré syndrome, CIDP. See p. 29.
 2. Charcot-Marie-Tooth dz: The most common hereditary neuropathies. CMT-1 is demyelinating, CMT-2 is axonal. Both start in the feet, usually before age 20, with weakness, numbness, and pes cavus.
 3. Cranial neuropathies: Important to distinguish central from peripheral neuropathies. See also individual nerves or sx.
  a. Cranial polyneuropathy syndromes:
   1) **Cavernous sinus syndromes:** See p. 41.
   2) **Basilar meningitis.**
   3) **Jugular foramen syndromes:** Variable compression of the lower four cranial nerves. Look for corticospinal signs or Horner's syndrome as evidence for brainstem compression.
   4) **Polyneuritis cranialis:** A variant of Guillain-Barré syndrome; see p. 29.
   5) **Myasthenia gravis:** See p. 63.
   6) **Botulism.**
  b. Bell's palsy:
   1) **H&P:** Pressure/pain behind ear, hyperacusis, decreased taste, subjective but not objective numbness. Unilateral face weakness including brow, eye closure (can see eye roll up). Examine eardrum to rule out Ramsay-Hunt syndrome (geniculate herpes, unrelated to the Ramsay-Hunt syndrome of myoclonus and spinocerebellar atrophy).

    2) **Rx:** Eye protection (drops during day, ointment and patch at night). Consider PO methylprednisolone within 24 h of symptom onset.

    3) **Tests:** If no improvement in 2 wk, consider Lyme Ab, CBC, ESR, CXR (to r/o TB, sarcoid, adenopathy), ACE, HIV, MRI, UBJ/SIEP if elderly.

4. Diabetic neuropathy:

  a. Types:

    1) **Polyneuropathy:** Distal, sensory > motor, axonal degeneration on EMG.

    2) **Autonomic neuropathy:** Gastroparesis, orthostasis, burning pain.

    3) **Diabetic amyotropy:** Asymmetric painful lumbosacral plexopathy.

    4) **Mononeuropathy:** e.g. pupil-sparing 3rd nerve palsy. Usually recovers.

  b. DDx: Tabes, amyloid (look for family history, paraprotein in blood or urine), spinal cord compression,....

  c. Rx: see "Neuropathic pain," p. 68, and "Diabetes mellitus," p. 162.

5. Plexopathies:

  a. Brachial plexopathy: See Figure 8.

    1) **H&P:** Sudden shoulder pain, worse with arm movement, then weakness of shoulder, arm, hand. Often with numbness on upper arm. Ask about previous viral syndrome; smoking history. Look for Horner's syndrome.

    2) **DDx of brachial plexopathy:** Pancoast tumor, postradiation therapy, DM, vasculitis, entrapment (p. 75), idiopathic brachial neuritis,....

    3) **Tests:** CXR, glucose, ANA, ESR; EMG (won't be positive < 3 wks after sx start).

    4) **Rx:** Steroids do not help idiopathic cases.

    5) **Prognosis:** Idiopathic cases usually start to recover in 4 wk; upper plexus may fully recover by 1 yr; lower plexus may take 2-3 yrs.

  b. Lumbosacral plexitis:

    1) **H&P:** Sudden leg pain, then weakness, paresthesias but little objective sensory loss. Straight leg raise may be positive, but there should be no back pain or exacerbation of pain by Valsalva maneuver. Pt. needs pelvic and rectal exams.

    2) **DDx:** Pelvic mass, postradiation therapy, DM, vasculitis, femoral neuropathy, radiculopathy,....

    3) **Tests:** Consider CEA, PSA, glucose, ANA, ESR, pelvic CT, EMG won't be positive < 3 wk after sx start, but is crucial to diagnosis: should see at least two spinal levels involved, with sparing of the paraspinal muscles.

    4) **Rx:** Steroids do not help.

    5) **Prognosis:** Pain gets better before strength; only slow, incomplete recovery.

6. Entrapment neuropathies and traumatic nerve injuries:

  a. H&P: Ask about repetitive activities, e.g. typing; comorbid dz, e.g. alcoholism, DM, hypothyroidism, acromegaly, arthritis, cancer; previous entrapments (consider hereditary neuropathy with pressure palsies). Light touch (cotton wisp) is often lost before pin prick (opposite to spinal cord injuries). Referred pain is common; e.g. pain above wrist from carpal tunnel syndrome.

b. **Brachial plexus trauma:** See diagram of brachial plexus, Figure 8.

 1) **Upper plexus lesion** = Erb-Duchenne palsy, often from trauma pulling head away from shoulder.

   a) **Motor:** Bellhop's tip position: internal rotation at shoulder, with elbow extension. Weak shoulder abduction and extension, weak biceps and triceps.

   b) **Sensory:** Numb over deltoid, radial forearm.

 2) **Lower plexus lesion** = Dejerine-Klumpke palsy; often from forced arm abduction, or lung apex tumor (Pancoast tumor; often with Horner's syndrome). See claw deformity similar to ulnar neuropathy, below.

c. **Common entrapment syndromes** (see also spinal level by nerve, p. 70)

 1) **Median nerve entrapment.**

   a) **Anterior interosseous nerve syndrome:** Branches just distal to elbow. Decreased flexion of D1-D2 causes weak pinch. <u>No</u> sensory loss.

   b) **Carpal tunnel syndrome:**
   - **H&P:** Tingling or numbness in D1-D4 (through medial but not lateral ring finger). Pain may radiate above wrist, but not to neck. Pain awakens pt. from sleep. Exam is not that sensitive. May see weak grip, thenar atrophy.
   - **Phalen's sign:** 60 sec of wrist flexion causes paresthesia.
   - **Tinel's sign:** tapping on wrist causes paresthesia.
   - **DDx:** Cervical radiculopathy, thoracic outlet syndrome, pronator teres syndrome, de Quervain's dz,....

 2) **Radial nerve entrapment**

   a) **Mid-upper arm compression:** (Saturday night or honeymoon palsy). See wrist and finger drop; no triceps weakness.

   b) **Forearm compression:** Finger drop without wrist drop. Consider surgery for entrapment.

 3) **Ulnar nerve entrapment.** Ulnar claw deformity: fingers 4 and 5 have metacarpal hyperextension with finger flexion.

   a) **Wrist vs. elbow compression:** Make a fist; if poor flexion of 4 and 5, then lesion is above wrist.

 4) **Thoracic outlet syndrome:**

   a) **Compression** of the brachial plexus by a cervical rib or elongated transverse process of C7. However, cervical ribs are common in normals. Maneuvers to look for obliteration of radial pulse have very low specificity.

   b) **Droopy shoulder syndrome:** Usually young women. Pulling down on arm worsens sx.

5) **Meralgia paresthetica:** Lateral femoral cutaneous nerve compression, often from weight change, causes thigh tingling.
6) **Peroneal nerve palsy:** From calf compression or long bedrest. See foot drop, steppage gait. Numb lateral calf and foot dorsum. Weak foot inversion suggests L5 root lesion. In trauma, anterior compartment syndrome, which requires <u>immediate</u> fasciotomy, can cause peroneal palsy.
7) **Tarsal tunnel syndrome:** Posterior tibial nerve.
   d. **Tests for compression:** Consider getting EMG if surgery is an option. EMG may be normal for the first 2-4 wk after onset of sx.
   e. **Rx of entrapment:** Splint, NSAIDS; consider surgery.

PSYCHIATRIC DISORDERS

A. **Emergencies:** When a patient becomes suicidal, violent, or attempts to leave the hospital after being declared incompetent. Be aware of regulations governing use of restraints.
   1. **Calm pt. down verbally.** Try hard. It may help to tell them that their behavior is frightening you and the rest of the staff.
   2. **Chemical restraint:** Pt. is more likely to accept oral meds if you offer a "choice" between oral and IM.
      a. **Oral:** Lorazepam 1-4 mg or haloperidol 5-10 mg.
      b. **IM:** Haloperidol 5 mg, lorazepam 2 mg, benadryl 50 mg IM.
   3. **Physical restraint:** Usually four-point "locked leathers." Consider five-point (e.g. straps across chest) for big young patients. Soft restraints may be enough for frail demented patients, but they usually have hidden reserves of strength and ingenuity. No one should be in physical restraints for more than a short time without sedation. Consider requesting sitters.

B. **Psychiatric mental status exam**
   1. **Appearance:** Disheveled, bizarre clothing choice (toga with gold eye shadow,...)
   2. **Behavior:** Cooperativity, restlessness,....
   3. **Speech:** Volume, rate, latency, prosody,....
   4. **Affect:** Restricted, labile, irritable, sad,....
   5. **Mood:** Screening questions—How are your spirits? How has your mood been? Do you enjoy yourself? What do you look forward to? Do you feel hopeless? When people feel like you do, they often think about hurting themselves; do you sometimes feel this way?
      a. **If suspect depression:** SIGECAPS questions—<u>S</u>leep change, <u>In</u>terest in activities decreased, <u>G</u>uilt, <u>E</u>nergy loss, <u>C</u>oncentration loss, <u>A</u>ppetite change, <u>P</u>sychomotor retardation, <u>S</u>uicidal thoughts. 4/8 strongly suggests depression, though strictly need 5.
      b. **If suspect mania:** DIGFAST questions— <u>D</u>istractibility, <u>In</u>judicious behavior (spending sprees, fights,.....), <u>G</u>randiosity, <u>F</u>light of ideas, <u>A</u>ctivity increased, <u>S</u>leep decreased, <u>T</u>alkativeness.
   6. **Thought content:** Suicidal or homicidal thoughts, ideas of reference, delusions (paranoia, guilt, somatic, obsessive, compulsive).
   7. **Thought process:** Looseness, tangentiality, thought blocking.
   8. **Perceptions:** Auditory, visual, or command hallucinations. Gustatory

or olfactory suggest temporal lobe epilepsy.

9. Mini-Mental Status Exam: Useful for quantifying change in mental status over time.

Max score (30)	MINI-MENTAL STATUS EXAM
	ORIENTATION
5	What is the year, season, date, day, month?
5	Where are we: state, county, town, hospital, floor?
	REGISTRATION
3	Name 3 objects: 1 sec to say each. Then ask pt. all 3. 1 point for each correct answer. Then repeat them until pt. learns all 3. Count trials, and record. ( )
	ATTENTION AND CALCULATION
5	Serial 7's. 1 pt for each correct. Stop after 5 answers. As an alternative, spell "world" backwards.
	RECALL
3	Ask for the names of the 3 objects repeated above. 1 pt for each correct.
	LANGUAGE
2	Name a pencil and a watch.
1	Repeat the phrase "No ifs, ands, or buts."
3	Follow a 3-stage command: "Take the paper in your right hand, fold it in half, and put it on the floor."
1	Read and obey the following: "Close your eyes."
1	Write a sentence.
1	Copy the design shown here:
	LEVEL OF CONSCIOUSNESS
	Assess along a continuum: alert, drowsy, stupor, coma

Table 17. The Mini-Mental Status Exam. (From *Psychiatry Res.*, Folstein, M.F. 1975;12:189-198, with permission from Elsevier Science.)

C. Anxiety disorder and panic attacks:

1. DDx: Cardiac or respiratory event, drugs (e.g. steroids, marijuana, cocaine), hyperthyroidism, labyrinthitis, temporal lobe epilepsy, mania.

2. Tests: TSH, consider EKG or ABG during an attack.

3. Acute rx: Alprazolam 0.5-1 mg, repeat after 30 min.

4. Chronic rx: SRIs or tricyclics (same doses as for depression, see p. 130), clonazepam, psychotherapy. Alternatives include buspirone or zolpidem.

D. Depression:
Depression is common, 10-15% incidence. Up to 50% in Parkinson's, Alzheimer's, stroke. Screen all your pts.

1. DSM-IV criteria for depression: Two weeks of depressed mood + 5/8 neurovegetative sx (SIGECAPS criteria; p. 76).

2. Affect: Patients who smile or laugh can still be depressed. Conversely, diseases like Parkinson's can give a false appearance of depression.

3. DDx of depression: Dementia, bipolar disorder, grief, malignancy (especially pancreatic cancer and brain tumor), Parkinson's dz, hypothyroidism, dysthymia (chronically depressed mood with only two SIGECAPS criteria),....

4. Rx of depression:

a. Drugs: See p. 130. Contraindications include a h/o mania, cardiac dz (avoid anticholinergic TCAs, try SRIs), dementia (avoid anticholinergic antidepressants), hypotension (try an SRI), angle-closure glaucoma, prostatic hypertrophy.

   b. Psychotherapy: Best in combination with meds.

   c. Electroconvulsive therapy:

     1) **Indications:** Especially good for refractory depression in the elderly. Good for catatonic depression. Epilepsy is not a contraindication. Stop any benzodiazepines or other anticonvulsants the day before.

     2) **Contraindications:** Brain tumor.

E. Catatonia: Sustained postures with waxy flexibility, often echolalia and automatic obedience. Responds to benzodiazepines.

F. Mania: More than 2 wk of euphoria + three of the DIGFAST criteria (p. 76), or irritability + 4 of the DIGFAST criteria.

   1. Acute rx: Benzodiazepines e.g. clonazepam, or neuroleptics.

   2. Chronic rx: Lithium or depakote; sometimes neuroleptics.

G. Obsessive-compulsive behavior:

   1. H&P: Ask about ritual touching, counting, checking, handwashing; hours per day spent on rituals. Distinguish between obsessions (thoughts) and compulsions (behavior).

   2. DDx: Also seen in degenerative dz, grief, Tourette's syndrome, anoxic encephalopathy, magnesium and carbon monoxide poisoning, Sydenham's chorea.

   3. Rx: Often treated with SRIs.

H. Organic personality change: Causes include focal lesions (trauma, strokes, tumors, epilepsy), degenerative dzs, drugs and toxins, infections (HIV, syphilis),....

   1. Frontal lobe damage:

     a. Orbitofrontal: Disinhibition.

     b. Frontal convexity: Apathy, poor sequencing, perseveration.

     c. Medial frontal: Akinetic, incontinent, leg weakness.

   2. Temporal lobe damage: Problems with memory, alternating restlessness and apathy, paranoia, Kluver-Bucy syndrome with hyperorality, hypersexuality.

I. DSM-IV personality disorders:

   1. Cluster A (odd or eccentric): Paranoid, schizoid (reclusive, detached), and schizotypal (bizarre, magical thinking).

   2. Cluster B (dramatic or emotional): Antisocial, borderline, histrionic, and narcissistic.

   3. Cluster C (anxious or fearful): Avoidant, dependent, obsessive-compulsive, and not otherwise specified (includes passive-aggressive, masochistic, etc.).

J. Hallucinations and delusions:

   1. DDx: Drugs, structural lesions, degenerative dz, complex partial seizures, sensory deprivation, psychotic depression or mania, schizophrenia (chiefly auditory hallucinations).

   2. Rx: Neuroleptics; consider zyprexa, rispiridol, or quetiapine to avoid extrapyramidal side effects.

K. Schizophrenia: Usually treated with neuroleptics.

   1. Organic disorders that can mimic schizophrenia: Hallucinogens, dementia, fluent aphasia, delirium tremens, diffuse CNS vascular dz (including lupus and syphilis), Huntington's dz, Wernicke-Korsakoff syndrome, endocrine dysfunction.

L. Schizoaffective disorder: Having traits of both schizophrenia and an affective disorder. Do not confuse with schizoid or schizotypal personality disorder (see above).

RADIATION THERAPY

A. Gray = 100 rads (1 centiGray = 1 rad)
B. Indications: Tumor; sometimes inoperable AVMs.
C. Doses:
    1. Brain: 6500-7500 cGy in 6-8 wks (5x/wk), usually 4000 cGy to whole brain + 2000 boost to tumor. 5% will get radiation necrosis; higher with proton beam therapy.
    2. Cord: For big (> 10 cm) field, usually use < 3.3 Gy in 42 days; small field < 4.3 Gy.
D. Side effects
    1. Acute: From edema. Increase steroids.
    2. Subacute: (Weeks to months). Lethargy from brain radiation therapy, Lhermitte's sign from spine radiation therapy.
    3. Late: (months to years).
        a. Presentations: Dementia, focal deficits, poor vision, endocrine abnormality.
        b. Causes: Radiation necrosis, pituitary insufficiency, new tumors (gliomas, GBM, meningiomas, nerve sheath tumors), radiation myelopathy (usually from cervical > thoracic radiation therapy).
        c. Tests: PET or SPECT to tell recurrent tumor from scar. PET has about 90% sensitivity and specificity.
        d. Rx: Both respond to surgery; XRT and chemotherapy for recurrent tumor only.
E. Stereotactic radiosurgery: Has long latency to obliteration.
    1. Indications: Best for lesions 2.5-3 cm, especially AVMs that are deep or in eloquent cortex. Also schwannomas (especially bilateral), pituitary adenomas, craniopharyngiomas, pineal tumors, metastases. Cavernous malformations are controversial.
    2. Methods:
        a. Gamma knife: Photons. Multiple focused sources.
        b. Linac: (Linear accelerator): photons.
        c. Proton beam: From cyclotron. Best for irregular lesions.
    3. Postop care: Anticonvulsants, analgesics, antiemetics.

SEIZURE

A. Status epilepticus: A seizure that lasts for more than 30 min, or seizures that recur for more than 30 min without regaining consciousness in between. This is an emergency.
    1. Initial assessment: ABCs (airway, breathing, cardiac), O_2 saturation, coma exam (see Coma and brain death, p. 24), EKG, IV access, draw labs.
    2. Initial Rx:
        a. Thiamine, glucose: 100 mg IV, 50% dextrose 50 ml, naloxone.
        b. Lorazepam (Ativan): 2 mg IV q2min x 5, or diazepam (Valium) 5

mg IV q3min x 4 while starting phenytoin load.

   1) **Pediatric dosing:** Diazepam 0.2 mg/kg IV at 1 mg/min, to max. of 10 mg. Or lorazepam 0.1 mg/kg IV under age 12, 0.07 mg/kg over age 12.

  c. Phenytoin (Dilantin): 1 gram IV over 20 minutes (or 18 mg/kg at 50 mg/min). Cardiac monitor; check BP q min. Consider fosphenytoin, p. 128, as an alternative.

   1) **Pediatric dosing:** 20 mg/kg IV at 0.5 mg/kg/min.

3. Full assessment: H&P (see below), intubate if necessary, check labs, stat head CT. Consider LP + Abx if pt. is febrile or has never seized before. Send phenytoin level 20 min after load. Consider emergent EEG if pt. is comatose, to rule out nonconvulsive status.

4. Second-line Rx: If seizures don't stop. Usually requires EEG monitoring, intubation and arterial line (see p. 189) for BP monitoring.

  a. Phenobarbital (Luminal): 20 mg/kg IV (100 mg/min) if still seizing after 40 min despite phenytoin and lorazepam.

  b. Pentobarbital (Nembutal): 5 mg/kg IV load if still seizing after phenobarbital. Titrate dose (0.3-9 mg/kg/h) to obtain 3-15 sec periods of burst supression on EEG.

  c. Midazolam (Versed): 0.2 mg/kg IV loading dose as alternative to phenobarbital/pentobarbital. Titrate dose (0.1-0.4 mg/kg/h) to get burst supression on EEG.

  d. Supportive care: Pressors if necessary. Cool patient if febrile. Stop anticonvulsant drip once a day to see underlying EEG rhythm.

5. Special cases:

  a. Partial status epilepticus: May be confused with tremor.

  b. Nonconvulsive status epilepticus: May present as coma or confusion, but usually there is focal motor activity such as rhythmic blinking. Nearly all patients in nonconvulsive status are known epileptics. A test of 1-4 mg lorazepam IV/SL/PO should cause improvement (also improves catatonia).

  c. Pyridoxine deficiency: Consider giving pyridoxine 1 g IV or more if pt. is on isoniazid.

B. Seizure H&P: Aura, behavior during seizure, postictal period, h/o previous seizures or status epilepticus, drugs tried, nocturnal tongue-biting or incontinence; febrile seizures as child, head injury, recent alcohol or other drugs, illness, sleep deprivation, relation to menstruation.

C. DDx of seizures: Syncope, myoclonus, tremor, jerking movements of bilateral pontine infarct, pseudoseizure, narcolepsy.

  1. Pseudoseizures: No abnormal EEG during seizure; thought to be "psychogenic," but not necessarily malingering. 50% of pts. with pseudoseizures also have real seizures at some point.

	Epileptic seizure	Pseudoseizure
Clonic limb mvt.	In phase bilaterally	Out of phase
Vocalization	"Epileptic cry" mid-seizure	Moans, screams, at start of seizure
Head turning	Unilateral	Violent side-to-side

Table 18. Differentiating epileptic and pseudoseizures.

D. Management of first seizure:
  1. **Causes of new-onset seizures:** Cerebral ischemia, bleed, trauma, mass, hydrocephalus, infection, toxin, metabolic, withdrawal (alcohol, benzodiazepine), overdose (cocaine, TCA, isoniazid), amyloid angiopathy, anoxia (usually doesn't respond to anticonvulsants), idiopathic.
  2. **Tests:** Consider head CT or MRI, LP, electrolytes (vigorous seizure alone can cause acidosis), Ca/Mg/phos, CBC (vigorous seizure alone can cause WBC), screen urine and blood for toxins, EEG (best with sleepdeprivation; photic stimulation, and hyperventilation), CXR to rule out lung primary tumor. Prolactin level elevation is unreliable evidence of a seizure.
  3. **Uncomplicated first seizure:** If pt. is young, healthy, with normal exam, you can skip emergent CT and LP, just get outpt. MRI + gadolinium, EEG. Give anticonvulsant until those results come back.
  4. **Hospital admission:** Consider admitting pts. with nonresolving change in their neuro exam, elderly pts. with first seizure (for more rapid tumor workup), alcoholics with active withdrawal.
  5. **Acute seizure rx:**
      a. **Benzodiazepines:** For alcohol withdrawal seizures, or if pt. seizes repeatedly. Lorazepam 2-4 mg IV/IM or diazepam 5-10 mg IV. Use only lorazepam in liver failure. Lorazepam has a slower onset but lasts longer (1 h vs. 20 min) than diazepam because it is less fat soluble. This is the opposite of their sedative effects.
      b. **Phenytoin:** Not for alcohol withdrawal seizures. Don't need to load it IV if patient is not actively seizing.
          1) **Oral:** 300 mg PO q3h x 3; then 300 mg qhs. Warn pt. of side effects: double vision, vertigo, fatigue.
          2) **IV:** 1g phenytoin over 45 min on cardiac monitor. If pt. is in status epilepticus, give it in 20 min. Painful.
      c. **Transition to chronic drugs:** Consider immediately starting a switch to another agent, if you think that would be a better long-term choice.
      d. **Discontinuing anticonvulsants after a single seizure:** It is usually safe to taper the drug after the cause of the seizures has been discovered and treated, or if EEG is normal and workup negative. In the latter case, chance of recurrence is about 30%.
E. Seizure classification by clinical type:
  1. **Generalized:**
      a. **Tonic-clonic** ("grand mal"): LOC with bilateral jerking, often preceded by aura. Often tongue-biting or incontinence, post-ictal confusion. A focal onset or Todd's (transient focal postictal) paralysis

suggests the seizure is secondarily generalized from a partial seizure.
- **b. Atonic** ("drop attacks"):
- **c. Absence** ("petit mal"): Usually in children; see p. 119.
- **d. Myoclonic epilepsy:** Usually in children; see p. 118.
2. **Partial** (focal, local): May become secondarily generalized.
   - **a. Simple** (no impairment of consciousness): May be motor, sensory, or autonomic, depending on site of focus.
   - **b. Complex** (impairment of consciousness): Often preceded by psychosensory aura. Seizure has confusion ± automatisms. Often from mesial temporal or frontal lesion.
F. **Management of chronic seizures.**
   1. **Causes of chronic seizure disorder (epilepsy):**
      - **a. Underlying defect:** Structural damage, genetic, metabolic.
      - **b. Precipitants of seizure:** fever; low anticonvulsants, Ca, Na, or blood sugar; sleep deprivation, or the acute causes listed above
   2. **Typical seizure, known epilepsy:** Pts. can leave emergency room as soon as they are back to baseline. They don't need a head CT unless they have head injury and nonresolving change in their neuro exam.
   3. **Rx. of seizure disorder:**
      - **a. Avoid precipitants:** Alcohol, sleep deprivation. Oral contraceptives may help perimenstrual seizures.
      - **b. Avoid driving:** Laws vary; it is typically illegal for pt. to drive for 6 months after a seizure.
      - **c. Anticonvulsants:** See p. 128. In general, increase levels of a single drug until seizures are controlled or until side effects are intolerable, before adding a second agent.

Seizure type	First-line agent	Second-line agent	AVOID
Partial or secondarily generalized	Carbamazepine > valproic acid	Phenytoin > phenobarbital	
Primary generalized	Valproic acid	Carbamazepine	Ethosuximide
Absence	Ethosuximide	Valproic acid	Phenytoin
Myoclonic	Valproic acid	Clonazepam	Phenyt., carbam.
Neonatal or febrile	Phenobarbital	Phenytoin	
Centrotemporal	Phenytoin	Phenobarbital	
Infantile spasms	Clonazepam	Steroids	
Lennox-Gastaut	Valproic acid	Lamotrigine	

Table 19. Choice of anticonvulsant.

- **d. In pregnancy:** See p. 188.
- **e. Epilepsy surgery:** To treat poorly controlled, disabling seizures after more than a year of failed aggressive medical management.
- **f. Discontinuing anticonvulsants:** Typically considered if patient hasn't had a seizure in 2 yr. May want to check EEG; chance of recurrence is higher if EEG is abnormal. See also p. 128, for taper regimens.
G. **Seizure prophylaxis:** In certain instances, patients should be on anticonvulsants even if they have never had a seizure. Consider prophylaxis in the following cases:
   1. **Brain tumor:** See p. 90. Usually not necessary, unless there is danger

of herniation, or it is a melanoma.

2. Post head injury: See Trauma, p. 89.

3. Intracranial hemorrhage: See p. 50. All pts with spontaneous subarachnoid hemorrhage should get an anticonvulsant; subdural and parenchymal bleeds are controversial; probably don't need prophylaxis.

4. Routine craniotomy: Consider 2 wk of anticonvulsant.

H. Proconvulsant drugs: The following may lower seizure thresholds in some pts.: some Abx (amphotericin B, β-lactams, fluconazole, isoniazid, metronidazole, praziquantel, zidovudine), anticholinergics, antihistamines, glucocorticoids, lithium, naloxone, narcotics (especially meperidine), neuroleptics, oxytocin, all stimulants, TCAs, X-ray contrast agents.

SENSORY LOSS

A. H&P: Patients use "numbness" to mean everything from tingling to paralysis. Ask about pain, paresthesias, hyperpathia. Look for dermatomal or individual nerve distributions, distal vs. proximal differences, spared modalities, graphesthesia, stereognosis, neglect to bilateral simultaneous stimulation. Associated signs: weakness, skin changes, cranial nerve abnormalities.

1. Hysterical numbness: Be suspicious of deficits that stop exactly at the midline, especially if a tuning fork is perceived differently on the two sides of the forehead. However, some patients may overgeneralize or misreport a real deficit, such as a crossed face and body numbness.

B. DDx:

1. Mononeuropathies and monoradiculopathies: Usually trauma or compression; consider also vasculopathy (e.g. from diabetes), zoster, leprosy.

2. Symmetric distal sensory loss ("stocking-glove"): Usually polyneuropathy from chronic illness or toxin.

3. Hemianesthesia: Damage to sensory cortex, thalamus, white matter.

4. Dissociated or crossed sensory deficits: Often from brainstem or spinal cord lesions; generally with other neurological deficits.

   a. Brainstem syndromes: See brainstem stroke syndromes, p. 23.

   b. Posterior column: Ipsilateral decreased position, vibration, stereognosis (but often bilateral involvement).

   c. Hemisection (Brown-Séquard syndrome): Ipsilateral decreased position and vibration; contralateral decreased pain and temperature. Little change in fine touch. Upper motor neuron signs beneath level of lesion.

   d. Central cord syndrome: Usually from syringomyelia (cavity near the central canal). Often begins cervically, with cape-like loss of pain and temperature sensation, then gradual spasticity and loss of light touch, sometimes facial or tongue weakness.

5. Paresthesias: Peripheral neuropathy or compression, peripheral vascular dz, spinal cord dz, metabolic disturbance, e.g. hypocalcemia or respiratory alkalosis, postherpetic neuralgia,....

SLEEP DISORDERS

A. Insomnia:

1. **H&P:** Ask about onset, trouble with initiating vs. maintaining sleep, drugs, movements in bed.

2. **DDx:** Pain, anxiety, depression, bad sleep hygiene, alcohol or tranquilizer dependence, medications (steroids, β-blockers,...), nocturnal movement disorders; occasionally sleep apnea or midbrain damage.

3. **Acute rx:**
   a. **Sedating antidepressants:** At these doses, these drugs are not antidepressant, but good for sleep induction; non-addictive.
      1) **Trazodone:** 25-50 mg PO qhs.
      2) **Doxepin:** 25-50 mg PO qhs.
   b. **Sedating antihistamines:** e.g. diphenhydramine 25-50 mg. Probably a little better than placebo for a day or two.
   c. **Benzodiazepines:** Try to avoid these, especially in elderly patients. If you must, use a short-acting one like lorazepam 0.5-1.0 mg.

4. **Chronic rx:** Stop caffeine, alcohol, and sleeping pills; retire and rise at same time every day, no reading in bed.

B. Excessive sleepiness:

1. **H&P:** Distinguish between excessive drowsiness and daytime fatigue from insomnia. Ask about sleep latency, daytime sleeping, medications, snoring, scratchy throat in am, cataplexy, sleep paralysis.

2. **DDx:** Sleep deprivation, depression, drugs, metabolic disorder.

3. **Tests:** Overnight sleep-EEG study.

4. **Sleep apnea:** Cessation of breathing during sleep.
   a. **Obstructive apnea:** If severe, can cause pulmonary hypertension, arrhythmia. Treat with d/c of sedatives, weight loss, nightly CPAP.
   b. **Central apnea:** From brainstem lesions, dysautonomias, neuromuscular dz. May require tracheostomy.

5. **Narcolepsy:** Lifelong disorder of REM sleep architecture.
   a. **Sx:** Frequent daytime sleep attacks, episodes of cataplexy (hypotonia), and more nonspecific signs of sleep deprivation, e.g. sleep paralysis, hypnagogic hallucinations.
   b. **Rx:** For sleepiness, stimulants, e.g. methylphenidate 5 mg q am and noon. For cataplexy, TCAs, e.g. imipramine 25 mg tid.

C. Nocturnal movement disorders:

1. **DDx:** Hypnagogic jerks (benign, single), nocturnal seizures (often at REM transitions),....

2. **Restless leg syndrome:** While resting but still awake, pt. feels an urge to move legs, often to relieve dysesthesias. Try clonazepam 0.5-2 mg, Sinemet 25/100 or 50/200 CR, or carbamazepine 200 mg.

3. **Nocturnal myoclonus:** While sleeping, pt. has rhythmic leg jerking that may awaken him. May occur in combination with restless leg syndrome. Try clonazepam.

D. Parasomnias:

1. **REM behavior disorder:** Loss of normal REM atonia— pt acts out his or her dreams. Associated with alcohol. Treat with safety precau-

tions, clonazepam 0.5-2 mg.
   2. Sleep-walking: Occurs during non-REM sleep. Try clonazepam.

SPINAL CORD

A. Acute cord compression: Any pt. with rapidly progressive spinal cord
   sx, especially involving bladder or bowel, should get a sensory and motor
   rectal exam, and an emergent spinal MRI. Consider dexamethasone 100
   mg IV push, emergent surgery or XRT. See also spinal tumors, p. 94.
B. Patients with back pain and known cancer: Assume cord compression
   until proved otherwise. See p. 94 for workup.
C. Terminology:
   1. Vertebral dz:
      a. Spondylosis = degeneration. "Cervical spondylosis" sometimes
         used as synonym for "stenosis."
      b. Spondylolisthesis = anterior subluxation.
      c. Spondylolysis = isthmic spondylolisthesis.
   2. Myelopathy: Myelopathy and myelitis refer respectively to damage
      to the spinal cord and inflammation of the spinal cord. Do not confuse
      with myopathy and myositis, which refer to muscle conditions.

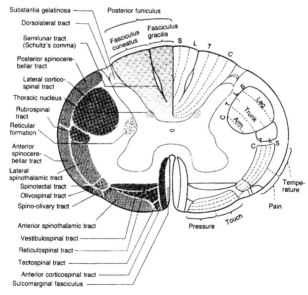

Fig. 2.7   Cross-section of spinal cord showing topography of ascending and
descending pathways and the somatotopic arrangement of their fibers.

Figure 9. The spinal cord in cross section. (From Duus P. *Topical Diagnosis in Neurology.* New York:Thieme, 1983: 49, with permission.)

D. History: Radiation of pain, triggers, numbness, weakness, incontinence, weight loss, IVDA, DM, previous surgery, trauma, litigation, degree of disability, associated depression. When neck pain, ask about chest pain, shortness of breath, radiation to jaw.

1. **Location:** Thoracic level suggests metastases.
2. **Character:** Burning, electric, aching.
3. **Precipitants:** Walking, sitting, squatting, leaning forward, coughing, time of day.
4. **Bladder changes:** Frequency, urgency, sensation during voiding, sexual function.
   a. **UMN lesion:** Bladder stretch reflex is disinhibited and spastic, so bladder is small and voids frequent.
   b. **LMN lesion:** Large retentive bladder, sometimes with overflow.
E. **Exam:** Check pain on palpation, range of motion, posture (anthropoid in stenosis), abdominal reflexes, clonus, pulses, atrophy, fasciculations, café-au-lait spots, Lhermitte's sign. Document exam carefully, especially if going to OR, to record presurgical deficit.
   1. **Straight leg raise (SLR):** for L5, S1 irritation. Pain during reverse SLR (extension) suggests L3 or L4 irritation.
   2. **FABER** (Flex-ABduct-Extend-Rotate): Put ankle on opposite knee; rotate knee toward exam table. Positive for hip dz and mechanical low back pain, but not for disc dz.
   3. **Psychiatric component:** Pt. has pain on simulated axial loading (push top of head), or can't tolerate SLR, but can sit/put socks on.
   4. **Bowel/bladder:** Check prostate, bulbocavernosus (finger in rectum, pull on penis or bladder catheter), cremaster, anal wink, percuss bladder, measure postvoid residual (if residual > 100 ml, leave catheter in). Any abnormality may be indication for emergent MRI.
   5. **Sensory lesions:** Look for sensory level, dissociation of sensory modalities. Pinprick is lost first (vs. peripheral nerve injury, where light touch is lost first). See Sensory loss, p. 83.
   6. **Conus medullaris vs. cauda equina compression:** The former is a cord lesion, the latter peripheral nerve. However, prognosis is similar, and sx often overlap.

	Conus medullaris	Cauda equina
Onset	Sudden, bilateral	Gradual, unilateral
Pain	Mild, bilateral	Severe, radicular
Bladder/bowel	Severe, early sx	Late sx
Sensory loss	Touch/pain dissociation, symmetric saddle distrib.	No dissociation; asymmetric distrib.
Motor loss	Mild, symmetric, may have fasciculations	Marked, asymmetric, + atrophy, fascics rare
Reflexes	Lose ankle but not knee jerk	May lose knee jerk too

Table 20. Distinguishing conus and cauda syndromes.

F. **DDx:** Tumor, trauma, disc herniation, epidural abscess, osteomyelitis, vasculitis, aortic dissection, cord embolus, bleed, transverse myelitis, spondylitis, carcinomatosis, Guillain-Barré syndrome, CIPD, schistosomiasis,....
   1. **Central cord syndrome:** Arms weaker than legs, decreased pain and

temperature sensation. LMN signs in some segments. Later, UMN signs below the lesion. Anterior spinal artery infarct can do this.

2. **Cortical vs. spinal or peripheral lesion:** Former has slow movements, latter has fast but weak movements.

3. **Disc herniation vs. spinal stenosis:**
   a. **Stenosis worse with walking,** better with leaning forwards.
   b. **Both worse with coughing** and Valsalva maneuver.
   c. **Stenosis causes brisk reflexes,** toes can be up. Disc herniation causes dropped reflexes.

4. **Paraparesis:** Consider spinal stenosis or mass, falx meningioma, spinal ischemia, thyrotoxic paralysis. Check orthostatic BPs.

5. **Tumor:** Pain worse lying/at night. Weakness usually legs first—not clear why there is usually sacral sparing. Position/vibration sense very sensitive for compression. Occasionally ataxia.

6. **Bilateral lumbosacral plexopathy:** In pelvic cancer, HIV,....

7. **Ankylosing spondylitis:** Get plain films of sacrum; HLA B-27 Ag.

8. **Leptomeningeal metastases:** See Brain tumors, p. 93.

9. **Thoracic outlet syndrome:** Either neural or vascular. Check pulses in different arm positions.

10. **Cervical cord contusion:** Usually after hyperextension with underlying stenosis or instability.

11. **Paget's dz.**

12. **Compression fracture.**

G. **Tests:**

1. **Spine MRI:** 24% of <u>asymptomatic</u> pts. have bulging disc; 4% have stenosis. Consider pain premedication. MRI useless if pt. has metal in back (e.g. previous surgery), but hip replacements are usually OK.
   a. **Screening sagittal view of whole spine:** If you suspect metastasis (30% have second metastasis).
   b. **Contrast:** If you suspect leptomeningeal dz or carcinomatosis, or if previous surgery and want to tell scar from disc.

2. **C-spine X-ray series** If recent neck trauma. Consider flexion-extension C-spine films, especially if transient quadriparesis after a neck injury, or if there is A-P pain.

3. **Lumbosacral X-rays:** Usually useless except if spine may be unstable; then get flexion-extension films.

4. **CT myelogram:** If MRI contraindicated, previous back surgery, or suspected CSF leak or obstruction.

5. **LP:** Can show high protein below CSF obstruction, because of pooling.

6. **Bone scan:** Not useful except as screen for infection or metastases all over. Rarely positive if plain films and ESR nl. Doesn't show myeloma.

7. **Blood:** Consider ESR, UBJ, SIEP, PSA, CA125, CEA.

8. **EMG:** If need to distinguish radiculopathy (nl nerve conduction velocity, but F-wave abnormal) from peripheral neuropathy. Denervation changes after disc occur 1-2 wk in paraspinous muscles; 2-5 wk in leg. Polyphasic renervation potentials start ~10 wk.

H. **Rx of back pain, cord injury:**

1. **Acute cord compression:** For trauma, use methylprednisolone proto-

col available in most ERs. Stat neurosurgery consult. Also see Spine tumors, p. 94.

2. **Cervical disc herniation:** NSAIDS, soft collar, physical therapy; consider surgery if myelopathy.
    a. **Home traction:** Kit available in surgical supply stories. 10-20 min qd, facing door, 6-8 lbs in sandbag. Head should be pulled 15 degrees forward, not back. Pressure on both occiput and mandible. Shouldn't hurt.
3. **Lumbar disc herniation:** NSAIDS, physical therapy; consider surgery if myelopathy. Bed rest rarely helps.
4. **Stenosis:** NSAIDS, physical therapy; surgery. Pt. can often tolerate exercycle more than other forms of exercise.
5. **Cervical cord contusion:** High-dose steroids, hard collar unless cervical instability already ruled out with C-spine X-ray (but don't flex/extend if there is a known cord contusion).

SYNCOPE

A. **H&P:** Try to find a witness.
    1. **Precipitants:** Exertion, stress, meals, alcohol, drug, cough, swallowing, urination, postural change, head movements, poor POs.
    2. **Sequelae:** Tonic/clonic movements, drowsiness, confusion, neurological changes, nausea, sweatiness, cold, incontinence, tongue biting, injury from fall, amnesia.
    3. **Exam:** Orthostatic BP and HR (immediate and delayed), BP in both arms, bruits (carotid, subclavian, supraorbital, temporal), heart exam. Look for trauma from fall. Stool guaiac.
B. **Causes:**
    1. **Cardiac:**
        a. **Arrhythmic:** AV block, sick sinus syndrome, long QT interval, pacer malfunction.
        b. **Obstructive:** MI, global ischemia,valve stenosis or dysfunction, PE, pulmonary HTN, aortic dissection, tamponade, left atrial myxoma,....
    2. **Vascular reflex:**
        a. **Vasovagal:** From fear, urination, Valsalva maneuver.
        b. **Orthostatic:**
            1) **Hyperadrenergic:** Volume depletion, varicose venous pooling, supine hypotension of late pregnancy (pressure on aorta).
            2) **ANS insufficiency:** Vasoactive or antidepressant drugs, neuropathies, spinal cord dz, paraneoplastic dz, parkinsonism.
        c. **Carotid sinus hypersensitivity:** A diagnosis of exclusion; can be elicited in 1/3 of normal old men.
            1) **Cardioinhibitory:** Common. Carotid sinus massage (see p. 169) causes sinus pause; blocked by atropine.
            2) **Vasodepressor:** Rare. Carotid sinus massage causes low SBP, blocked by epinephrine, not atropine.
    3. **Neurological:** Vertebrobasilar TIA (carotid TIAs almost never cause syncope), seizure, subclavian steal, NPH.
    4. **Metabolic:** Hypoxia, hypoglycemia, hyperventilation.

    5. Psychiatric.

C. Tests: Rule out risk of sudden death; reserve further testing for recurrent syncope only.

    1. Cardiovascular: EKG for MI, LV hypertrophy, arrhythmia. Consider echocardiogram, Holter monitor, ETT; perhaps signal-averaged EKG, tilt test, electrophysiological stimulation.

    2. Blood: CBC, electrolytes, toxin screen, CPKs.

    3. CXR: If suspect CHF, PE (± ABG, V/Q scan), pericardial effusion, mitral stenosis.

    4. Neurological tests: (Low yield unless focal deficit or bruits): CT, carotid and cranial ultrasound, EEG.

    5. Carotid sinus massage: See p. 169. Cardiac pause of > 3 sec, or SBP drop < 30 points with sx, or more than 50 without, is abnormal. Abnormal response confirms cause only if it reproduces sx, and other causes are excluded.

D. Orders: VS q shift with orthostatic BPs, guaiac all stools, cardiac monitor, IV fluids slowly, keep BP > 140. For autonomic insufficiency, see p. 61.

TRAUMA

A. Types of injury: See p. 147 for CT appearance of head trauma.

    1. Intracranial hemorrhage: See p. 50.

    2. Concussion: Brief LOC with no parenchymal abnormalities on CT.

    3. Contusion: Predominantly gray matter, after blunt head trauma.

    4. Shear injury (diffuse axonal injury): Seen especially after deceleration injury.

    5. Contrecoup injury: Seen when the brain is thrust against the skull opposite from the primary blow.

    6. Dissection: Of carotid or vertebral artery.

    7. Skull fracture.

B. Indications for head CT: Focal deficit, anticoagulation, significant LOC, drug intoxication. Usually don't need to get a CT in pts. with very brief LOC and no focal neurological signs.

C. Exam: Note exact time of exam, amount and time of last sedation.

    1. General: Vital signs and pattern of respiration. Palpate head for skull fractures, facial fractures. Look for lacerations, racoon eyes, Battle sign (bruise behind ear). Fundi (papilledema, hemorrhage, retinal detachment). Blood in nose or ears; CSF leak (see p. 18). Listen for bruits over eyes, carotids. Look for evidence of spine trauma.

    2. Quick neurological exam:

        a. Assess alertness; coma exam (see p. 24).

        b. R/o spine injury:

            1) **Rectal:** Including anal wink and bulbocavernosus.

            2) **Sensory:** Pinprick all 4 limbs and trunk; touch major dermatomes C4, C6-8, T4, T6, T10, L2, L4-S2. Vibration and proprioception for posterior columns.

            3) **Motor:** In more detail than just noting "moving all extremities."

            4) **Cerebellar exam:** If pt. cooperative.

D. Rx:
1. **Consider neurosurgery consult:**
2. **Spinal cord trauma:**
   a. **Methylprednisolone:** Must be given within 8 h of injury. 30 mg/kg initial IV bolus over 15 min; then wait 45 min, then 5.4 mgh/kg/h for 23 h.
   b. **Blood pressure and temperature control:** May be very labile.
   c. **Nasogastric tube:** For paralytic ileus.
   d. **Bladder catheter:** To avoid bladder distension.
3. **Head trauma:**
   a. **Indications for seizure prophylaxis:** If there is any blood in head, Glasgow Coma Scale (GCS) < 10, penetrating brain injury, or significant alcohol history, give anticonvulsant x 1 wk. If pt. needs craniotomy, give x 6 mo.
   b. **Indications for mannitol:** Evidence of herniation (e.g. dilated pupils) or local mass effect (e.g. hemiparesis), or sudden deterioration. Hypotension is a relative contraindication.
   c. **Indications for intubation:** GCS < 7, inability to protect airway (e.g. from maxillofacial trauma), need for hyperventilation to reduce ICP.
   d. **Admission orders for moderate head injury:** GCS 9-13.
      1) **Neurological checks:** q1-2h.
      2) **Activity:** HOB up 30-45°.
      3) **Diet:** NPO until alert or no risk of surgery; then clear liquids. NS + 20 mEq KCl/L at 75 ml/h.
      4) **Meds:** Mild analgesics and antiemetics. Avoid phenothiazines, which lower seizure threshold.

TUMORS, BRAIN

A. H&P: Focal deficit (68%,usually weakness), HA (54%—if worse lying flat, suggests hydrocephalus), seizure (26%—suggests frontal/temporal, slow growing), N/V (suggests posterior fossa), personality change (suggests midline frontal), papilledema.
B. DDx of brain tumor: Abscess, bleed, infarct, demyelination, radiation necrosis,....
C. Tests: MRI + contrast (p. 148), or CT + contrast (p. 148) if pt. unstable, or question of hemorrhage. Brain biopsy vs. resection. Consider workup for unknown primary tumor (usually CXR, mammogram, chest and abdominal CT), LP to rule out leptomeningeal spread.
D. Rx of brain tumor: See also specific tumor types, below.
1. **Treat edema:** Consider one or more of the following:
   a. **Dexamethasone:** Bolus 10 mg IV, then 4 mg q6h. Taper after radiation therapy. If you suspect CNS lymphoma, try to withold steroids until biopsy.
   b. **Fluid restrict:** 1200 ml qd, no free water.
   c. **Mannitol:** 50-100 grams IV, then 25-50 grams q6h to keep osmolality 305-310.
2. **Neurosurgery:**
   a. **Resection:** Unless inaccessible, multiple foci, or very radiosensi-

tive. Consider surgery for all posterior fossa tumors > 3 cm even if there are other metastases.

   b. **Biopsy:** In situations where full resection is inadvisable but a tissue diagnosis is necessary.

   c. **CSF access procedures:** See p. 67. Ventriculostomy or VP shunt for hydrocephalus, Ommaya reservoir for intraventricular chemotherapy.

3. **Radiation therapy:** Consider 2-3 days steroids before beginning XRT, to decrease swelling, especially in posterior fossa lesions.

4. **Chemotherapy:** Regimens change often. See p. 133 for side effects.

5. **Seizure prophylaxis:** There is little need for prophylaxis in patients who have never seized, except if there is a risk of herniation, or with hemorrhagic metastases. Metastases in the cerebellum or deep subcortical areas rarely cause seizures.

E. **Prevalence:**

1. **Metastases:** 30-50% of all brain tumors. 15% of pts. with cancer have brain metastasis as presenting complaint. 10% present with seizures.

2. **Primary intracranial tumors:** Astrocytomas (including GBM) 58%, meningiomas 20%, pituitary tumors 14%, acoustic schwannomas 7%, oligodendrogliomas 4%, craniopharyngiomas 3%, lymphomas 1%.

F. **Metastases to CNS:**

1. **Most common source:** Usually carcinoma >> sarcoma or lymphoma.

   a. **Intracranial metastases:** lung > breast > melanoma > primary never found (9%) > renal > colon. Prostate is very rare.

   b. **Dural, epidural, skull metastases:** breast, prostate.

   c. **Leptomeningeal metastases:** See p. 93.

2. **Tumors most likely to have brain metastases:** Melanoma (40%).

3. **Metastases likely to bleed:** Adenocarcinomas (renal > thyroid > GI, pulmonary, breast), melanomas, choriocarcinomas.

4. **Number:** On CT, 50% are solitary, 20% have two metastases.

   a. **Solitary metastases:** Always consider biopsy, because 10% are benign, even if the patient has another known primary.

   b. **Multiple metastases:** Consider resection of the dominant, symptomatic lesion.

5. **Location:** 90% are supratentorial, 10% cerebellar (50% of cerebellar metastases are pelvic/GI).

6. **Prognosis for brain metastases:**

   a. **No rx:** 4 wk survival.

   b. **Steroids alone:** 8 wk.

   c. **Steroids + radiation therapy:** 3-6 mo (most die of other cause).

   d. **Surgery:** up to a year.

G. **Gliomas:** Include glioblastomas, astrocytomas, oligodendrogliomas, ependymomas.

1. **Brainstem gliomas, cerebellar astrocytomas, ependymomas:** Mostly pediatric; see p. 120.

2. **Astrocytomas:**

   a. **Grading:** WHO grades I-III are replacing older 1-4 schemes. (Roughly, 1 = benign astrocytoma, 2 = low-grade malignant astrocytoma, 3 = anaplastic astrocytoma, 4 = glioblastoma = GBM. 3 and 4 are also called malignant gliomas.)

Grade	Scan Findings	Survival	Rough pathol.	Treatment
I	Mass	Benign	Pilocytic	Surgery
II	Mass	7-10	Atypia	Surgery
III	Enhancement	~2	Mitoses	Surg/chemo/XRT
IV	Ring en-	<1	Necrosis or	Surgery/XRT/
	hancement		vasc. prolif.	chemo

Table 21. WHO astrocytoma grading.

    b. Recurrence: ~90% are at original site. Some white-matter spread (e.g. "butterfly" glioma across callosum). Metastases rare.

    c. Rx of astrocytoma: Surgery, radiation therapy (see p. 79), alkylating agents e.g. PCV (procarbazine, CCNU, vincristine).

  3. Oligodendrogliomas: > 50% frontal; 20% bifrontal. Often present with seizures. Often calcified. More chemosensitive than astrocytomas.

H. Meningiomas: (20% of intracranial primaries). Arise from the arachnoid. Indolent. 8% are multiple, higher in type 1 neurofibromatosis.

  1. DDx: Includes prostate or breast metastasis to bone.

  2. Scans: "Lightbulb" enhancement, attached to meninges. Often calcified, with adjacent hyperostosis.

  3. Rx: Surgery usually curative, often bloody. May need pre-op angio ± embolization, to see if blood supply is from ECA or ICA, confirm dx (prolonged homogeneous tumor blush), and assess venous sinus occlusion. Radiation therapy, for partially resected meningiomas, is controversial.

I. Pituitary tumors:

  1. H&P:

    a. Secretory tumors: Sx of hormonal excess, e.g. Cushing's syndrome, acromegaly, or galactorrhea.

    b. Nonsecretory tumors: Sx of mass effect, e.g. bitemporal field cuts, headache, hypopituitarism, invasion of cavernous sinus.

    c. Pituitary apoplexy: An emergency. See sudden headache, visual deterioration, diplopia, and drowsiness. From bleed into tumor. Requires immediate surgery to preserve vision.

  2. DDx: Suprasellar mass, pituitary infarct or apoplexy, inflammation.

  3. Tests: MRI with gadolinium and thin cuts through sella (see p. 151), adrenal function (see p. 162), thyroid function (see p. 163), prolactin, follicle-stimulating and luteinizing hormones, estradiol in women, testosterone in men, growth hormone if there is acromegaly.

  4. Rx:

    a. Surgery: Usually transsphenoidal or pterional (see p. 67). Indications include apoplexy, acromegaly, Cushing's syndrome, macroadenomas, prolactinomas with PRL < 500 ng/ml (chance of normalizing PRL > 500 is low) or unresponsive to bromocriptine.

    b. Medical:

      1) **Bromocriptine:** For prolactinomas, start 1.25-2.5 mg qd; add additional 2.5 mg qd every 3-7 d as necessary. Usual dose is 5 - 7.5 mg qd. Some growth hormone tumors respond to higher

doses of bromocriptine, e.g. 20-30 mg qd. Max. dose is 100 mg qd.

  2) **Octreotide:** For growth hormone-secreting tumors. Very expensive. Side effects include GI disturbance, gallstones. 100-200 μg SQ q 8h.

  3) **Adrenal, thyroid, and sex hormone replacement therapy.**

  c. **XRT:** Not routinely used. Side effects include hypopituitarism, optic nerve damage, lethargy, diplopia, and pituitary apoplexy.

J. Vestibular schwannomas: AKA acoustic neuromas (although they are not neuromas and usually arise from the vestibular nerve, not the acoustic), and acoustic neurinomas. Benign, cerebellopontine angle tumors.

  1. **H&P:** Hearing loss, tinnitus, imbalance; later headache, facial numbness, weakness, or diplopia. Look for signs of neurofibromatosis. Bilateral vestibular schwannomas are pathognomonic for neurofibromatosis type II.

  2. **DDx:** Meningioma (often nerve V involvement before VII, calcification on CT) or other tumor.

  3. **Tests:** MRI with thin cuts, or CT with contrast. Audiological testing may help establish a baseline for post-surgical comparison.

  4. **Rx:** Usually surgery; stereotaxic radiosurgery is sometimes used for recurrence. Expect significant but usually transient post-op nausea and ataxia. Facial nerve dysfunction can be treated by hypoglossal-facial anastomosis.

	Good surgical candidate	**Poor surgical candidate**
Tumor < 3 cm	Good hearing → surgery	Observation[1]
	No hearing → observation[1]	
Tumor > 3 cm	Surgery	Surgery or radiosurgery

Table 22. Management of vestibular Schwannomas. [1]Observation = repeat neurological exam and imaging q 6 mo x 2 years, then annually if stable. If exam deteriorates or growth is > 2 mm/yr, consider surgery or radiosurgery.

K. Lymphomas

  1. **Rx/prognosis:** Untreated, 4 mo. Traditional XRT: 15 mo. High-dose methotrexate (experimental): 4 yr. No role for surgery.

  2. **In HIV:** Chief differential is toxoplasmosis. If there are multiple lesions, don't biopsy; give 2 wk empiric toxoplasmosis therapy and look for response. If none, consider XRT. Many HIV pts. are too ill to tolerate chemotherapy.

L. Leptomeningeal metastases: Can be the presenting problem before primary is known. Most common in leukemia, lymphoma, breast cancer, lung cancer.

  1. **H&P:** Synchronous signs or sx at multiple sites in brain, cranial nerves, or spinal cord. Often back pain or postural headache.

  2. **Tests:**

   a. **CT or MRI:** To r/o mass before LP. Communicating hydrocephalus suggests leptomeningeal dz. A scan with contrast may show meningeal enhancement.

   b. **LP:** Do cytology for malignant cells (80% sensitive after three

LPs). Send at least 3 ml. Cells degrade quickly—don't let them sit.

   3. Rx: Response depends on primary tumor. Most breast cancers and lymphomas respond, as do about 30% of lung cancers, and 20% of melanomas. Untreated pts. usually die within weeks.

      a. XRT: Irradiate symptomatic areas. Often given with dexamethasone.

      b. Chemotherapy: Usually intrathecal methotrexate. Consider Ommaya reservoir.

      c. Ventriculoperitoneal shunt: For symptomatic hydrocephalus.

TUMORS, SPINE

A. H&P, DDx: See Spinal cord, p. 85.

B. Leptomeningeal tumors: See Brain tumors, p. 93.

C. Back pain in a pt. with cancer: Assume spinal cord compression until proven otherwise.

   1. Neurological deficit on exam:

      a. Dexamethasone: 100 mg IV bolus

      b. Emergent MRI or myelogram.

         1) **Tumor and > 80% stenosis:** give emergent XRT, consider surgery. Continue dexamethasone 96 mg qd; taper as tolerated.

         2) **Tumor and < 80% stenosis:** nonemergent XRT ± surgery.

         3) **No tumor:** symptomatic rx.

   2. No neurological deficit: Get plain spine films.

      a. If abnormal x-ray: with > 50% collapse of a vertebral body, or pedicle erosion, get emergent MRI and proceed as above.

      b. If normal xray: Get nonemergent MRI.

D. Types of spine tumor: Most are benign, and compress rather than invade

   1. Extradural: (55%)

      a. Metastases: Common. Consider lung, breast, prostate, lymphoma.

      b. Primary: Rare. Chordomas, neurofibromas, osteoid osteomas, osteoblastomas, aneurysmal bone cysts, vertebral hemangiomas.

   2. Intradural extramedullary (40%): Schwannomas, meningiomas, neurofibromas, lipomas.

   3. Intramedullary (5%): Astrocytomas (30%), ependymomas (30%), miscellaneous.

E. Tests:

   1. MRI: Emergent in any case of suspected spinal cord compression. Multiple lesions are common, so request longitudinal scout of entire spine. For MRI appearance of spinal cord tumors, see p. 152. Consider CT-myelogram in patients who can't have MRI.

F. Rx:

   1. Blood pressure: Very labile with cord lesions, especially to pain. Overtreating BP, e.g with nifedipine, can cause hypotension.

   2. Acute cord compression rx: Goal is to prevent progression, although deficit can sometimes reverse if it is of recent onset.

      a. Dexamethasone: 100-mg bolus, then 24 q6h. In breast cancer and lymphoma, steroids kill tumor, as well as decreasing edema and pain.

      b. Neurosurgery consult: Emergent.

1) **Indications:** Decompression, tissue diagnosis, displaced bone or ligament, unstable spine, or relapse at previously irradiated site. May reverse paraplegia.

2) **Relative contraindications:** Very radiosensitive tumor (myeloma, lymphoma), total paralysis > 24 h.

  c. **Radiation therapy:** Within 12 h. See below. 50% of nonambulatory pts. walk, but paraplegic ones remain so.

3. **Nonemergent cord compression management:**

  a. **Dexamethasone** 10 mg q6h.

  b. **Radiation therapy:**

    1) **Dose:** 300 rad fractions x 10 = 3000 rads. Higher dose causes transverse myelitis. Need to simulate and plan field carefully if window may overlap previous radiation therapy area.

    2) **Contraindications:**

      a) **Radioresistant tumor:** e.g. thyroid cancer, renal cancer, sarcoma.

      b) **Bone fragment:** If bone, not tumor, is compressing cord, pt. needs surgery, not radiation therapy.

      c) **Previous radiation therapy in same region:** Can't get radiation therapy twice in same field (unless pt. has only a few months life expectancy) because too much radiation therapy itself will cause paralysis.

  c. **Chemotherapy:**

    1) **Prostate metastases:** Start flutamide several days before starting lupron—latter has temporary agonist effect and can cause swelling with acute cord compression.

    2) **Lymphoma.**

    3) **Breast metastases:** Chemotherapy occasionally helps.

URO-NEUROLOGY

A. Bladder detrusor and internal sphincter:

1. **Parasympathetic:** Acetylcholine from S2-S4 via pelvic nerve constricts bladder via muscarinic receptors.

2. **Sympathetic:** Norepinephrine from L2-L4 via hypogastric nerve constricts sphincter via α-receptors. There are β-receptors on the bladder.

B. External sphincter: Voluntary control via S2-S4.

C. H&P: Often a poor correlation between sx and urodynamic findings.

1. **Autonomic dysreflexia:** <u>Urgent</u>. In pts. with spinal cord injury above L2, bladder distension or catheterization can trigger acute hypertension, bradycardia, anxiety, and headache. Treat promptly with nifedipine 10 mg SL, and sit the pt. up.

2. **Frequency or urgency:** From high fluid intake, urinary tract infection, partial outlet obstruction (prostate, diaphragm), upper or lower motor neuron lesion, psychogenic.

3. **Urinary retention:** From drugs (anticholinergics, opiates, anesthetics), pain, prostate, lower motor neuron lesion, bladder-sphincter dyssynergia, obstruction.

4. **Incontinence:**

  a. **Stress:** Often from bladder suspension defect or sphincter injury.

   b. Overflow: Dribbling, small volumes, big painful bladder. Causes
      are those of urinary retention, above.
   c. Confusional: Varying volumes, usually shameless.
D. Upper vs. lower motor neuron lesions.

	UPPER MOTOR NEURON	**LOWER MOTOR NEURON**
Bladder	Small, spastic, low PVR	Large, flaccid, high PVR
History	Urgency, trouble starting, wet at night	Strains to empty fully, wet or dry at night.
Bulbocavernosus	Present	Absent
Causes	Bilateral frontal lesion, cord lesion above T12	Anesthetics, neuropathy, ALS, cauda equina lesion
Treatment	Decrease bladder tone with anticholinergics or adrenergics	Increase bladder tone with cholinergics or antiadrenergics; self-catheterization

Table 23. Distinguishing upper and lower motor neuron lesions.

E. Urodynamic findings and rx:
   1. **Flaccid bladder:** Detrusor hyporeflexia, poor voiding. Treat with
      catheterization. Try cholinergics e.g. bethanechol (Urecholine), 10-50
      mg bid-tid. Avoid cholinergics in COPD, PUD, CAD, hyperthyroid-
      ism.
   2. **Spastic bladder:** Detrusor hyperreflexia, poor storage. Try anticho-
      linergics, e.g. oxybutinin (Ditropan), 5 mg bid-tid.
   3. **Spastic sphincter:** Detrusor-sphincter dyssynergia. Spinal cord le-
      sions above the sacral level can leave just the sphincter spastic. The
      bladder eventually dilates, but secondarily. Treat with catheterization,
      anticholinergics, or prazosin (an anti-α_1-adrenergic, 1 mg bid-tid).

VASCULITIS, CNS

	CNS	PNS	Muscle	Other organs	C3,C4	Tests	Biopsy
Polyarteritis nodosa	30	60	50	Kidney, heart	Down	RF, HBs-Ag	Muscle, nerve
Allergic granulomatosis	25	70	20	Lung	Up	Eosinophilia, igE	Muscle, nerve
Temporal arteritis	10	30	30	Polymyalgia	Up	ESR, alk phos, HLA-DR3, DR4	Temp Artery
Takayasu arteritis	40	/	<5	Great vessels	nl	Possibly ESR, HLA A10, B3, MB3, DR4	Arteries
Wegener's granulomatosis	25	15	/	Resp., Urogenital	Up	ANCA, HLA-DR2	ENT
Lymphomatoid granulomatosis	35	25	/	Lung, skin	nl	Lymphocytosis with leukopenia	Skin, lung
Hypersensitivity angiitis	10	20	10	Skin, kidney, joints	nl	Eosinophil count, IgE, IgA	Skin
Lupus erythematosus	60	10	10	Skin, joints, heart	Down	ANA, anti-ds-DNA, HLA-B8, -A15	Skin
Rheumatoid arthritis	<5	10	50	Joints	Up	RF	Joints
Scleroderma	<5	10	90	Skin, esophagus, joints	nl	RF	Skin
Mixed connective tissue dz	<5	90	90	Joints	Down	ENS Ab	Skin
Sjögren's syndrome	30	10	10	Eye, ENT (sicca)	nl	Schirmer's test	Pelvic rim
Thromboangiitis obliterans	?	—	—	Peripheral vessels	nl	Anti-elastin Ab	Salivary gland
Moya-moya syndrome	100	—	—	None	nl	HLA -AW24, -BW46, -BW54	Temp Artery
Sneddon's syndrome	100	—	—	Skin (livedo racemosa)	nl	Antiphospholipid Ab	—
Cogan's syndrome	?	—	—	Eye, ear	nl	ESR, CSF, HLA-BW17	Skin
Isolated CNS angiitis	100	—	—	None	nl	—	Skin
Behçet's syndrome	30	—	—	Aphthous ulcers, eye	C9 up	CSF, HLA-B5, -B12, -DR7	Brain

Table 24. Vasculitic syndromes.

VENOUS SINUS THROMBOSIS, CNS

A. **H&P:** HA 78%, papilledema 50%, seizure 40%, variable confusion, cranial nerve deficits, uni- or bilateral cortical signs, seizures. Variable time course. Can look like pseudotumor cerebri.

B. **Tests:**
   1. **MR venogram:** The test of choice. True angiogram usually not necessary.
   2. **Standard MRI:** Not sensitive. After day 5, standard MRI may show increased T1 and T2 signal along sinus.
   3. **CT:** Not sensitive. See focal hypodensity or petechial blood; can look like metastases. Small ventricles. Without contrast, the triangular "delta" of the sagittal sinus looks dense. If contrast given, can sometimes see empty delta sign, or gyral and falx enhancement.
   4. **CSF:** Usually normal; sometimes see decreased protein or increased RBCs.

C. **Rx of venous thrombosis:** Heparin, even if hemorrhagic infarct. Then warfarin x 2-3 mo. Consider thrombolysis. Mannitol and steroids. Phenytoin only if seizure.

D. **Prognosis:** Good; 75% have complete recovery.

VERTIGO

A. **History:** Try to distinguish between vertigo (illusion of movement or spinning) and dizziness (lightheadedness, a feeling that one might faint). Ask about suddenness of onset, HA, tinnitus, hearing decrease, other cranial nerves, gait, trouble controlling limbs, length of episode, LOC, change in vision, N/V, worse when stand/stoop/turn neck, h/o trauma, anxiety, hypo- or hyperglycemia, or hypertension.

B. **Physical exam:** Orthostatic BPs, bruits, hearing (see p. 45), eye exam, tympanic membranes; consider Romberg test, postural reflexes, hyperventilation x 3 min, calorics (see p. 189).
   1. **Bárány's test:** Have a bucket handy if pt. is nauseous. On a stretcher, bring pt. suddenly back from a seated position to supine with the head turned fully to the right. Have pt. keep eyes open, and watch for nystagmus and vertigo for at least 1 minute. Repeat with head to the left.

C. **DDx:** R/o dizziness from cardiac problem, bleed, panic, hypoglycemia; poor balance from movement disorder, sensory deficits, or weakness.

D. **Central vertigo:**
   1. **H&P:** Less sudden onset (or if sudden, with HA), less nausea, continuous sx independent of posture, usually no hearing loss.
      a. **Nystagmus:** All varieties of nystagmus including vertical.
      b. **Side of sx:** Falling and nystagmus are to same side, that of the lesion (vs. peripheral nystagmus, which is to opposite side).
      c. **Bárány's's test:** No latency to nystagmus, it lasts > 30 sec, no habituation. Nystagmus can go in different directions from same head position.
   2. **Causes of central vertigo:** Brainstem lesion, cerebellar lesion (especially PICA territory including flocculonodular lobe), acoustic

schwannoma. Phenytoin or barbiturates. Can see central vertigo in migraine or complex partial seizures. Multiple sclerosis may cause poor balance; rarely true vertigo. Vertebral dissection.

E. Peripheral (vestibular) vertigo:

  1. **H&P:** Often sudden, positional, with severe nausea, tinnitus, or decreased hearing.

     a. **Nystagmus:** Horizontal or rotatory nystagmus in only one direction.

     b. **Side of sx:** Sx are worse with bad ear facing down. Nystagmus (fast phase) is to opposite side of bad ear; past-pointing and falling are to same side.

     c. **Bárány's's test:** 2-20 sec latency to nystagmus; habituates in ~30 sec and on repeated testing.

  2. **Causes of peripheral vertigo:**

     a. **Drug-induced:** Alcohol, Abx, furosemide, quinidine, quinine, aspirin. Phenytoin and barbiturates cause vertigo centrally, not peripherally.

     b. **Benign positional vertigo:** Drugs don't work well. Try the Epley maneuver, followed by desensitization: tilt head x 30 sec 5x every few hrs.

     c. **Menière's dz:** Decreased hearing, ear fullness, tinnitus usually present. Attacks last minutes to hours, recur weeks to years. Try clonazepam 0.5 mg bid, meclizine 25 q6h, diuretics, or strict salt restriction.

     d. **Vestibular neuronitis:** Usually young, sudden, not recurrent, post-viral. No decreased hearing or tinnitus.

     e. **Other infections:** Chronic otitis media, herpes zoster oticus, syphilis (usually bilateral),....

WEAKNESS

A. See also: Neuromuscular disorders, p. 62.

B. Terminology: Paresis is partial; plegia or paralysis is complete.

C. H&P: Numbness, pain, distal vs. proximal, bowel and bladder function, injuries, diurnal or exercise-induced fluctuation, tone, reflexes, atrophy, fasciculations, etc.

  1. **Muscle strength grading scale:**

     0: No contraction.

     1: Flicker of contraction.

     2: Active movement, but can't resist gravity.

     3: Active movement against gravity.

     4: Active movement against resistance.

     5: Normal strength.

D. Upper motor neuron vs. lower motor neuron weakness: Both may be flaccid initially, but UMN lesion (corticospinal, pyramidal) usually develops spasticity and hyperreflexia; reflexes should be depressed in LMN lesion. May see fasciculations in LMN lesion; EMG will show fibrillations only after a few weeks. Dexterity is preferentially affected by upper motor neuron corticospinal lesion.

  1. **Spasticity:** An exaggeration of stretch reflexes, causing velocity-

dependent, "clasp-knife," rigidity, flexion dystonia, and flexor spasms, hyperreflexia.

    a. DDx: Extrapyramidal rigidity, muscle spasms,....

    b. Rx: Muscle relaxants (see p. 139). Physical therapy. Orthopedic procedures to release contractions.

E. Bulbar vs. pseudobulbar palsy:

    1. Bulbar palsy: Lower motor neuron flaccid lesion of lower cranial nerves. Decreased gag.

    2. Pseudobulbar palsy: Spastic, upper motor neuron lesion. Hyperactive gag. Causes include ALS, MS, and bilateral cerebral strokes. In the latter two, there is often "pseudobulbar affect": excessive, inappropriate laughing and crying.

F. Hemiparesis: Ipsilateral arm and leg. Typically from corticospinal damage. Look for other signs, e.g. neglect, cranial nerve abnormalities, to localize further.

G. Monoparesis: Single limb. May have a peripheral cause as well as central.

H. Paraparesis: Both legs. Usually spinal cord; look for sensory level. But consider falx meningioma or bilateral ACA infarcts.

I. Proximal, distal, or generalized weakness:

    1. Severe or quickly progressive quadriparesis: Consider high cervical or brainstem lesion, Guillain-Barré syndrome, botulism.

    2. Slowly progressive: Consider neuropathies, neuromuscular dz.

    3. Fluctuating weakness: Consider myasthenic syndromes, TIAs, hyper- or hypokalemic periodic paralysis.

    4. Generalized weakness in the ICU: Mnemonic for DDx is MUSCLES: Medication, Undiagnosed neuromuscular disorder, Spinal cord damage, Critical illness polyneuropathy, Loss of muscle mass, Electrolyte disorders, Systemic illness.

CHILD NEUROLOGY

DEVELOPMENT
A. H&P:
1. **History:** Problems or drug use in pregnancy, weeks gestation, Apgars, birth weight, postnatal problems, developmental milestones (see Table 26), school performance. For adolescents, try to ask about drugs and sexual activity with parents out of the room.
2. **General exam:** Head circumference (see growth curves, p. 109), eye exam, face and limb morphology, skin (café au lait, ashleaf, palmar creases), and cardiovascular exam. In infants, fontanelles (see p. 107), skull, and base of the spine.
3. **Neurological exam:** See primitive reflexes and developmental milestones, below.
   a. **Infants:** Alertness, posture, spontaneous movements, cry pitch and volume, pupil responses, ability to track a face, orientation towards noise, reflexes (see Table 25), response to pinch. Assess tone (premature infants are normally hypotonic).
      1) **Supine:**
         a) **Hypertonic:** Arched back, more than a few beats of clonus, asymmetric tonic neck reflex that is obligate or present after age 6 mo.
         a) **Hypotonic:** Frog-legged and little spontaneous movement.
      2) **Traction response:** Pull the infant from supine to sitting.
         a) **Hypertonic:** Persistent leg extension.
         b) **Hypotonic:** Head lag, no compensatory leg flexion.
      3) **Horizontal suspension:**
         a) **Hypertonic:** Back extension.
         b) **Hypotonic:** Infant drapes over your hands.
      4) **Vertical suspension:** Hold baby under armpits.
         a) **Hypertonic:** Scissoring of legs with plantar ankle flexion.
         b) **Hypotonic:** Head droops; baby slips through your fingers.
   b. **Older children:** Toddlers may be examined better on a parent's lap. Use toys to engage them; watch movement during spontaneous play.
B. Normal development:
1. **Primitive reflexes:**

Reflex	Appears by	Gone by (mo)
Gag	32 wk gest.	Persists
Suck	34 wk gest.	4
Palmar grasp	34 wk gest.	6
Plantar grasp	34 wk gest.	10
Tonic neck—incomplete (asymmetric)	34 wk gest.	4
Moro (arms, legs extend when head falls supine)	34 wk gest.	3
Automatic stepping when upright on table	35 wk gest.	2
Crossed adductor	35 wk	7
Extensor plantar response (Babinski)	Birth	10
Placing (when baby upright & foot brushes table)	1 day	2
Asymmetric tonic neck reflex[1]	2-3 wk	4-6
Landau (head, trunk, leg extension while prone)	3 mo	24

[1] If you turn baby's head, ipsilateral arm extends, contralateral arm flexes. A sustained tonic neck reflex is always abnormal: baby should stop posturing after a few sec. of your holding the head deviated.

Table 25. Primitive reflexes.

2. Developmental milestones:

Age	Gross motor	Fine motor	Language	Social
2 mo	Lifts chest off table	Follows object past midline	Responsive smile	Recognizes parent
4 mo	Rolls over	Moves arms in unison to grasp	Orients to voice	Enjoys looking around
6 mo	Sits unsupported	Grasps with either hand, transfers	Babbles	Recognizes strangers
9 mo	Crawls, pulls to stand	Pincer grasp, holds bottle	Understands no	Explores, plays pat-a-cake
12 mo	Walks alone	Throws objects	Uses 2 words besides dada/mama	Imitates, comes when called
18 mo	Runs	Feeds self with spoon	Knows body parts	Copies doing tasks, plays w/ others
24 mo	Walks up and down stairs alone	Turns single pages, removes clothes	Uses 2-word sentences, follows 2-step commands	Parallel play
3 yr	Pedals tricycle	Dresses partially, draws a circle	Uses 3-word sentences, plurals	Group play, shares toys
4 yr	Hops, skips	Can button, catches ball.	Knows colors, asks questions	Tells "tall tales"
5 yr	Jumps over low obstacles	Ties shoes, spreads with knife	Prints first name, asks word meanings	Plays competitively, follows rules

Table 26. Developmental milestones.

C. Intelligence quotient: IQ = (mental age/chronological age)x100. For adults, count chronological age as 16.

Degree of mental retardation	IQ	Mental age as adult
Dull normal	80-90	—
Borderline	70-79	—
Mild (educable)	55-69	9-11
Moderate (trainable)	40-54	5-8
Severe	25-39	3-5
Profound	< 25	< 3

Table 27. Degrees of mental retardation.

D. Normal patterns of myelination: Best evaluated by T1-weighted MRI for the first 4 months of life, T2-weighted thereafter. In general, myelination progresses caudal to rostral, central to peripheral, and dorsal to ventral. Because there is no gray-white differentiation in infants, it is easy to miss small amounts of edema.
   1. **At birth:** Central cerebellar white matter, superior and inferior cerebellar peduncles, brainstem, and thalamus.
   2. **By 1 month:** Corticospinal tracts, pre- and postcentral gyri, optic nerves and tracts.
   3. **By 3 months:** Middle cerebellar peduncles, optic radiations, and posterior limb of the internal capsule.
   4. **By 8 months:** Anterior limb of the internal capsule, corpus callosum, centrum semiovale, and subcortical U-fibers.
   5. **By 18 months:** Nearly adult appearance except for the peritrigonal region posterior to the occipital horns.
   6. **By 20 years:** Peritrigonal region is myelinated.
E. Progressive developmental delay or regression:
   1. **H&P:** Earlier trauma to nervous system, family history, consanguinity? Child abuse or neglect? A good general exam as well as neurological exam and head circumference. Look especially at skin, eyes, viscera (murmurs, hepatomegaly), dysmorphic features, growth failure.
   2. **Causes:** Consider hydrocephalus, tumors, autism, epilepsy, infections, toxins, abuse, and metabolic disorders.
       a. Gray vs. white matter dz?
          1) **Gray matter dz:** See personality change, seizures, cognitive decline, early EEG changes. Causes include tumors, severe epilepsy, ceroid lipofuscinosis, Heller's syndrome, Lesch-Nyhan dz, neuroaxonal dystrophy.
          2) **White matter dz:** See corticospinal sx, blindness, focal neurological deficits. Causes include progressive hydrocephalus, childhood MS, leukodystrophies, Alexander's dz, Canavan's dz, galactosemia, Pelizaeus-Merzbacher dz.
       b. Peripheral as well as central nervous system dz? Suggests lysosomal storage disorders; mitochondrial disorders.
       c. Other organs involved besides nervous system? Suggests aminoacidurias (see p. 112), neurocutaneous syndromes (see p. 116), TORCH infections (see p. 111), hypothyroidism, chronic toxin exposure.
   3. **Tests:**
       a. Blood: Electrolytes, CBC, lactate, liver function tests, lead levels.

    b. Neuroimaging: Look for hydrocephalus, focal lesions, atrophy, diffuse white matter change. Compare with normal progression of myelination, above.

    c. Other: Consider LP, metabolic tests (see p. 112).

F. Static developmental delay:

  1. DDx: Slowly progressive congenital disorders. Look for developmental regression, other systemic findings, peripheral neuropathy, family history.

  2. Cerebral palsy: Generic name for static encephalopathy, usually from prenatal rather than perinatal factors. Classified by motor findings.

    a. Spastic hemiplegia: (Arm and leg). Usually from developmental malformation or stroke. Usually normal intelligence, sometimes seizures.

    b. Spastic diplegia: (Legs >> arms). Usually from prematurity. Intelligence may be near normal; seizures rare. May need orthopedic rx of spasticity.

    c. Spastic quadriplegia: Usually from severe diffuse brain injury. Severe seizures and mental retardation are common.

    d. Athetoid: From hypoxia, cerebellar or basal ganglia lesions, kernicterus.

  3. Perinatal events:

    a. H&P: Maternal risk factors and delivery. Poor alertness, periodic breathing, hypotonia, seizures. Bulging fontanelles and signs of high ICP in severe hemorrhage.

    b. Term newborns:

      1) **Hypoxic-ischemic encephalopathy (HIE):** Acute total asphyxia injures thalamus and brainstem more; prolonged partial asphyxia injures cerebral cortex and white matter more. Alertness may improve between 12 to 24h of age and then deteriorate over the next 72h. Severe HIE causes mental retardation, spastic quadriparesis, and seizures, but mild HIE resolves within 2 d without sequelae.

      2) **Other:** Stroke, hemorrhage, etc.

    c. Premature infants:

      1) **Periventricular leukomalacia:** (PVL). Presumed to be from HIE. In premature newborns, this mostly affects subcortical white matter, causing spastic diplegia quadriplegia, or visual impairment. Severe HIE also causes mental retardation and microcephaly. PVL can be shown, after 1-2 wk, with CT or MRI.

      2) **Periventricular-intraventricular hemorrhage:** (PIVH). A germinal matrix hemorrhage, probably the effect of transient hypertension on vessels previously weakened by ischemia. Occurs in about 25% of newborns weighing < 2 kg, within the first 4 d.

        a) **Tests:** Head ultrasound. Should be performed as a screen in all newborns < 32 wk gestation, and in symptomatic newborns > 32 wk. Follow PIVH with serial US—10% will develop hydrocephalus.

      b) **Prevention:** Avoid premature birth. Avoid blood pressure fluctuations: complete paralysis of vented newborns, rapid volume expansion.

      c) **Management:** Continue BP control; treat hydrocephalus with drugs that decrease CSF production (e.g. mannitol, acetazolamide), ventriculostomy, or ventriculoperitoneal shunt.

4. **Structural malformations:**

  a. **Neurulation disorders:** e.g. encephaloceles, myelomeningoceles. When spinal, AKA spina bifida. The defect should be surgically closed within the first week or two of life. Hydrocephalus requiring VP shunt usually develops because of associated aqueductal stenosis.

  b. **Midline malformations:** e.g. holoprosencephaly (undivided anterior brain), septo-optic dysplasia.

  c. **Migration disorders:** e.g. schizencephaly (brain cleft from partial defect in neuronal germinative zone), lissencephaly (agyria), pachygyria (few gyri), polymicrogyria.

  d. **Differentiation disorders:** e.g. microcephaly, megalencephaly, neurocutaneous disorders, corpus callosum aplasia, Aicardi's syndrome (callosal agenesis with chorioretinal lacunae, vertebral defects, and infantile spasms in a girl), colpocephaly (enlarged occipital ventricular horns), congenital vascular malformations and tumors, porencephaly (cerebral cavity), hydranencephaly (severe bilateral porencephaly).

  e. **Cerebellar malformations**

    1) **Chiari malformation:** See also p. 147 for radiological appearance of tonsillar herniation. Sx range from headache to sx of cerebellar and brainstem compression.

      a) **Type I:** Cerebellar tonsils herniate below the foramen magnum.

      b) **Type II:** Cerebellar vermis, fourth ventricle, and medulla are below the foramen magnum. Usually with myelodysplasia and lumbar myelomeningocele.

      c) **Type III:** Brain displaced into a myelomeningocele. Rare.

    2) **Dandy-Walker malformation:** Vermis hypoplasia with fourth ventricle cyst and hydrocephalus, from blocked foramen of Magendie. Both the fourth and lateral ventricles must be shunted.

  f. **Myelination disorders.**

  g. **Arachnoid cysts:** Seen in 4% of normals; only 20% are symptomatic, usually from secondary hydrocephalus.

5. **Chromosomal defects:** e.g. trisomies, translocations, deletions, mosaicism.

  a. **Down syndrome:** (trisomy 21). 1/1000 live births.

    1) **General features:** Short, dysmorphic, simian crease, cardiac, thydroid, GI problems, increased risk of leukemia.

    2) **Neurological features:** Hypotonia, mental retardation, early Alzheimer's dz, cervical narrowing and risk for atlantoaxial

subluxation, seizures in 10%, nystagmus and sluggish pupils, hearing loss.

    b. Fragile X syndrome: See p. 120.

6. Gene disorders: Delay may be static or progressive (see p. 103).

7. Maternal diseases and toxins: e.g. TORCH infections, p. 111, fetal alcohol syndrome, complications of labor and delivery.

8. Postnatal insults: e.g. infections, malnutrition, toxins, cerebrovascular events, trauma, neglect.

EYES AND VISION

A. Nystagmus: See p. 42. Congenital nystagmus is often not noticed in infants, and thought to be acquired. It is sometimes associated with poor acuity.

    1. Spasmus nutans: Nystagmus with head nodding and abnormal head position. Onset 6-12 mo, lasts 1-2 yr, improves spontaneously.

B. Oculomotor palsy:

    1. H&P: Babies > 3 mo old should have conjugate gaze and good fixation. See p. 39 for exam. You'll probably need something more interesting than your finger to get a 2-year-old to track.

    2. Causes: See p. 39 for causes also seen in adults (tumor, aneurysm, thrombosis, etc.). Causes seen primarily in children include

        a. Infantile botulism: Hypotonia with big, sluggish pupils, autonomic dysfunction. May see ptosis without opthalmoplegia. Associated with eating honey. Unlike adult form, spores colonize gut. Antitoxin and antibiotics do not help.

        b. Congenital palsies: Duane's syndrome (poor ab- or adduction with globe retraction), Möbius' syndrome (bilateral 6th and 7th palsies), Brown's syndrome (congenitally short superior oblique muscle), congenital myasthenia.

        c. Infection: e.g. meningitis, Gradenigo syndrome (petrous inflammation).

        d. Kearns-Sayres syndrome: See p. 58.

        e. Ophthalmoplegic migraine: Sx begin during or just before a migraine, but may last up to 1 mo. Oculomotor nerve is affected in 80%.

C. Strabismus: Nonparalytic ocular misalignment. If constant and persistent, child will often fixate only with one eye, develop amblyopia (loss of acuity) in the other, and have no complaint of diplopia.

    1. H&P: If misalignment is fixed, test EOM monocularly to r/o paralysis. If it is intermittent, perform alternating cover test, p. 40. Test acuity, fundus exam.

    2. Rx: Alternate patching of the eyes. Corrective surgery. Botulinum toxin has recently been tried.

D. Vision:

    1. H&P: In babies, test pupillary, red, and blink reflex; have them track your face at a distance of approximately 30 cm. Babies over 3 mo should have a visual grasp reflex, but it is hard to test before 6 mo. Look for abnormal eye movements, structural abnormalities such as cataracts, fundal lesions, microphthalmia.

2. **Tests:** Visual evoked responses should be present by 30 wk gestation, and mature at 3 mo.
3. **Causes:** See p. 37 for causes also seen in adults (retinal ischemia, optic nerve or cortical lesions, etc.).
   a. **Acute:** Carotid dissection, ICH, hysteria, migraine, optic neuropathy (demyelinating, ischemic, toxic), pseudotumor cerebri, trauma.
   b. **Subacute or chronic:**
      1) **Compression:** Tumor, aneurysm, AVM, inflammatory mass.
      2) **Cataracts:** Genetic, intrauterine drug exposure (chlorpromazine, steroids, sulfonamides) or infection (mumps, rubella, syphilis), prematurity, endocrine abnormalities, trauma, postnatal varicella. Remove cataracts before 3 mo to prevent amblyopia.
      3) **Hereditary optic atrophies:** Sometimes isolated. Multisystem involvement is most often mitochondrial dz.
      4) **Tapetoretinal degeneration:** Usually disorders of carbohydrate or lipid metabolism, and associated with dementia, neuropathy, and ataxia.
      5) **Other:** Congenital optic nerve hypoplasia, coloboma (an embryonic retinal defect), Leber's congenital amaurosis (unrelated to the mitochondrial disorder of Leber's hereditary optic neuropathy), dislocated lens, corneal clouding (e.g. in mucopolysaccharidosis and Fabry's dz).

HEAD CIRCUMFERENCE ABNORMALITIES

A. **H&P:** Maternal history (toxins, infections, hypoxia), family head sizes. Get pt's prior head sizes. Rule of thumb for normal growth rate in premature infants: 1 cm/wk; 1-3 mo: 2 cm/mo; 3-6 mo: 1 cm/mo; 6-12 mo: 0.5 cm/mo.
   1. **Head circumference:** Largest measurement around forehead and occiput excluding ears. For a normal baby, it is approximately the crown-rump length. Abnormal = more than 2 SD above mean, circumference out of proportion to height and weight, or upward deviation of growth curve over time (crossing curves)
   2. **Head shape:** Frontal bossing suggests hydrocephalus, lateral bulging suggests SDH.
   3. **Fontanelles:** Posterior and sphenoid fontanelles closes by 2-3 mo, mastoid fontanelle by 1 yr, anterior fontanelle by 1.5-2.5 yr.
   4. **Ophthalmoscopic exam:** Look for papilledema, retinal bleed.

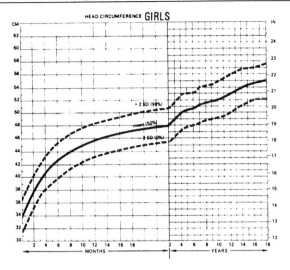

Figure 10. Head circumference, girls. (From Neilhaus G. *Pediatrics*, 1968;41:106, with permission.)

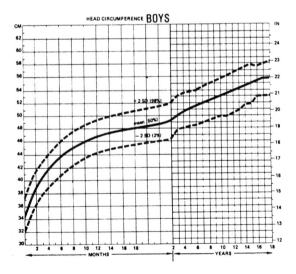

Figure 11. Head circumference, boys. (From Neilhaus G. *Pediatrics*, 1968;41:106, with permission.)

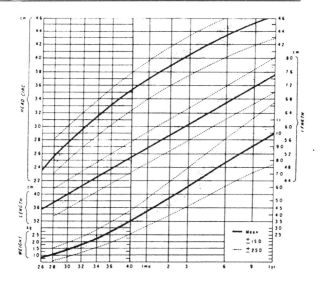

Figure 12. Fetal and infant head circumference, weight, and length. (From Lerner AJ. *The Little Black Book of Neurology*, 3rd ed. St. Louis: CV Mosby, 1995:65, with permission.)

B. Tests: CT, MRI, or ultrasound. Genetic and metabolic evaluation if microcephaly.

C. Causes of microcephaly: Genetic, intrauterine infections (CMV, toxoplasmosis, rubella), toxins (alcohol, anticonvulsants), asphyxia, metabolic disorders, radiation (especially 4-20 wk gestation).

D. Causes of macrocephaly: Hydrocephalus, SDH, hydranencephaly, megalencephaly.

E. Craniosynostosis:
  1. **H&P:** Deformed skull, firm pressure on either side of affected suture fails to cause movement. Look for other facial or body dysmorphisms; developmental delay.
  2. **Causes:** Premature fusion of sutures, failure of brain growth. Little evidence that it can be caused by shunting for hydrocephalus.
      a. **Sagittal synostosis:** Most common type, has long, boat-shaped skull with keel-like ridge.
      b. **Coronal synostosis:** If unilateral, affected forehead is flat or concave, and normal eye falsely appears to bulge. Can cause amblyopia.
          1) **Crouzon's syndrome:** Coronal synostosis plus midface hypoplasia. Hydrocephalus is rare.
          2) **Apert's syndrome:** Coronal synostosis plus syndactyly. Hydrocephalus is common.
      c. **Metopic synostosis:** Pointed forehead with midline ridge. Often with 19p chromosome abnormality and mental retardation.

   d. Lambdoid synostosis: Flattened occiput. If unilateral, causes rhomboid skull with bulging ipsilateral forehead.
   3. **DDx:** "Lazy lambdoid syndrome" (positional flattening from decreased mobility), congenital torticollis (causing baby always to lie on same side.
   4. **Rx:** Surgery.
F. **Hydrocephalus:**
   1. **H&P of active hydrocephalus:**
      a. **Hydrocephalus before cranial sutures close:** Cranium grows faster than face does, bulging fontanelles, irritability, N/V, poor head control, engorged scalp veins, Macewen's sign (cracked pot sound when percussing over dilated ventricles), 6th nerve palsy, upgaze palsy (see dorsal midbrain syndrome, p. 23), hyperactive reflexes, apneic spells.
      b. **Hydrocephalus after cranial sutures close:** Headache, papilledema, N/V, ataxia, 6th nerve palsy, upgaze palsy.
      c. **Entrapped 4th ventricle:** Sometimes seen with chronic shunting of lateral ventricles after infections. Headache, lower cranial nerve palsies, decreased alertness, ataxia, N/V.
   2. **Differential diagnosis of hydrocephalus:** Macrocrania (from rickets, chronic hemolysis, osteopetrosis), megalencephaly, hydranencephaly, benign external hydrocephalus (asymptomatic enlargement of subarachnoid space, with large head size).
   3. **Causes of hydrocephalus:** Either noncommunicating (obstructive), or communicating (decreased absorption, or rarely increased production, of CSF). Hemorrhage may cause hydrocephalus by either mechanism.
      a. **Congenital** (70%): Chiari II malformation, aqueductal stenosis, Dandy-Walker malformation, X-linked hydrocephalus.
      b. **Hemorrhagic** (15%): Post-intraventricular, post-subarachnoid. Common in premature infants.
      c. **Mass lesion** (11%): Often tumors around the aqueduct, e.g. medulloblastoma. Colloid cyst can intermittently block foramen of Monro. Because there is no gray-white differentiation in infants, it is easy to miss small amounts of edema.
      d. **Postinfectious** (8%): Purulent or basilar meningitis, cysticercosis.

HEADACHE IN CHILDREN

A. **See:** Headache (adult), p. 43, Ophthalmoplegic migraine, p. 106.
B. **H&P:** How much school is missed? Does it stop them from playing, or watching TV? Visual changes? Very young children may have only paroxysmal vomiting with or without paroxysmal vertigo. Check for stiff neck, papilledema, head circumference, tooth and ear infection, cerebral bruits (common, but should not be asymmetric), heart murmur.
C. **Causes:** See p. 43. In very young children, consider also occipital seizures (rare).
D. **Rx of migraine:** Similar to adults.
   1. **Acute rx:** Consider an NSAID + promethazine 1 mg/kg PO. Sumatriptan 6 mg SC has been safely used in school-aged children; divide the dose in half for smaller ones. Sumatriptan nasal spray may re-

place injections.

2. **Prophylaxis:** For children who miss school more than once a month. Try propranolol 0.5-1.0 mg/kg bid (asthma, diabetes, and depression are contraindications), or cyproheptadine 2-4 mg PO bid-tid. Consider also TCAs (monitor serum level and QT interval) or valproic acid.

INFECTIONS, CNS

A. **Meningitis:** See also meningitis in adults, p. 47.

1. **H&P:** Infants show nonspecific irritability or somnolence, fever, cyanosis, high-pitched cry, poor feeding, sometimes a bulging fontanelle or seizures. Before 1 yr of age, there is usually no meningismus; after that, you may see HA, stiff neck, Kernig's or Brudzinski's sign. Look for rash, mouth, ear lesions.

2. **DDx:** Mass lesion, including abscess, toxic exposure,....

3. **Tests:** CBC, electrolytes, blood cultures. LP, usually with prior head CT. See Table 3, p. 18, for CSF findings. Never delay empiric Abx— LP can be done up to 2 h after first dose without destroying culture results.

4. **Rx:** If you suspect *H. influenza* or there is high ICP, give dexamethasone 0.15 mg/kg IV q6h x 4 d. Respiratory precautions if you suspect *N. meningitidis*.

Patient	Likely pathogen	Antibiotic
Pre-term + low wt. neonate	Staph., gram-neg. bacilli, group B strep, *E. coli, L. monocytogenes*	Vancomycin 15 mg/kg IV q6h + ceftazidime 50-100 mg/kg q8h
0- 3 mo	Group B strep., *E. coli, L. monocytogenes*	Ampicillin 50 mg/kg IV q8h + ceftriaxone 50-100 mg/kg IV q12h
3 mo - 18 yr	*N. meningitidis, S. pneumo., H. influenzae.*	Ceftriaxone 50-100 mg/kg IV q12h + vancomycin 10 mg/kg IV q6h

Table 28. Empirical antibiotics for meningitis in infants and children. Adjust on the basis of C+S. (Adapted from Quagliarello VJ, Sheld WM. *N Engl J Med.* 1997;336:708, wieth permission.)

B. **TORCH infections:** Acronym for the major nonbacterial infections of neonates: Toxoplasmosis, Others (especially syphilis), Rubella, Cytomegalovirus, and Herpes simplex. All are acquired transplacentally except herpes, which the fetus catches in the birth canal.

1. **Toxoplasmosis:**
   a. **H&P:** Signs of diffuse cortical and subcortical lesions. Cataracts, microphthalmia. Sometimes liver, marrow, lung, muscle, and heart problems.
   b. **Tests:** Cerebral cortex and periventricular necrosis and calcification on CT; watch for hydrocephalus. Toxoplasma-specific IgM is often negative. CSF may show lymphocytosis, high protein, and trophozoites.
   c. **Rx:** Spiramycin, pyrimethamine, and sulfadiazine to infected mother and baby during the first year.

2. **Rubella:** Congenital rubella syndrome occurs when the fetus is infected < 20 wk gestation.
   a. **H&P:** Mild cases are normal at birth, then show CNS and ocular deficits, deafness, and heart dz. Severe cases have low birth

weight, liver failure, petechiae, cataracts, deafness, heart dz, microcephaly, bone lesions, and low platelets. Infected infants are highly infectious.
   - **b. Tests:** Viral culture of throat and urine. Serum rubella IgM.
   - **c. Rx:** Symptomatic.

3. **Cytomegalovirus:**
   - **a. H&P:** Only 10% of infected newborns are symptomatic at birth (liver failure, petechiae, microcephaly, periventricular calcifications, chorioretinitis). Of the 90% who are asymptomatic, 10% will later get deafness or microcephaly.
   - **b. Tests:** Urine culture.

4. **Herpes simplex:**
   - **a. H&P:** Local oral or opthalmic lesions (both may be <u>absent</u>), meningitis, or disseminated HSV with hepatosplenomegaly, DIC, renal failure, and encephalitis.
   - **b. Tests:** CSF is consistent with viral meningitis. Throat, urine, and stool cultures.
   - **c. Rx:** 14 d of acyclovir; do not wait for culture results to start.

METABOLIC DISEASES

A. **See also:** Progressive developmental delay, p. 103.
B. **H&P:** Progressive neurologic deterioration with recurrent unexplained ataxia, spasticity, altered consciousness, vomiting, acidosis; or mental retardation in the absence of major congenital brain abnormalities.
C. **Tests:** Electrolytes, glucose, ABG, ammonia, lactate, urine ketones, urine colorimetric tests (ferric chloride, DNPH, reducing substances, nitroprusside, CTAB Berry spot). Consider carnitine, serum and urine amino acids, urine organic acids, full ophthalmological exam, CT or MRI, skeletal films for bone age and defects, lysosomal enzyme studies, tissue biopsy.
   1. **Isolated ketosis:** Suggests maple syrup urine dz.
   2. **Ketosis and acidosis:** Organic acidopathy, lactate/pyruvate disorders.
   3. **Lactic acidosis:** Lactate/pyruvate or mitochondrial disorders; hypoxia, sepsis, liver or renal failure, DM.
   4. **Hyperammonemia:** Urea cycle disorders (without ketosis), organic acidopathies, Reye's syndrome, liver failure.
   5. **No ketosis, acidosis, or hyperammonemia:** Nonketotic hyperglycinemia, sulfite oxidase deficiency; peroxisomal, lysosomal, or fatty acid disorders.
D. **Causes:** The entries below focus on disorders for which prompt rx is essential.
E. **Abetalipoproteinemia:** (Bassen-Kornszweig dz). Infants have steatorrhea, ataxia, retardation, retinitis pigmentosa, low cholesterol, acanthocytes. Responds to vitamin E and special diet.
F. **Aminoacidurias:**
   1. **Homocystinuria:** Autosomal recessive defect in cystathione synthase causes accumulation of sulfur metabolites.
      - **a. H&P:** Normal at birth. The neurological sx are from strokes. Frequently mentally retarded, with psychiatric disorders. Also see skin and eye problems. Adult heterozygotes are also at risk for strokes.

     b. Rx: Pyridoxine 250-1000 mg qd, a methionine-restricted diet supplemented with cystine and betaine.

  2. Maple syrup urine dz: Autosomal recessive defect in branched-chain amino acid metabolism (valine, leucine, isoleucine).

     a. H&P: Normal at birth; sweet-smelling urine. Within a week get opisthotonos, intermittent increased muscle tone, irregular breathing. If untreated, severe retardation and spasticity; may die in infancy.

     b. Tests: Urine ferric chloride test; serum amino acids.

     c. Rx: Diet restricted in branched-chain amino acids. If started in first 2 wk of life, most children develop normally. However, they are vulnerable to sepsis.

  3. Phenylketonuria: Autosomal recessive defect of phenylalanine hydroxylase (converts phenylalanine to tyrosine).

     a. H&P: Normal at birth, vomiting and irritability by 2 mo, mental retardation by 4-9 mo; later seizures and imperfect hair pigmentation.

     b. Rx: Phenylalanine-restricted diet. If started early, children develop normally.

G. Hyperammonemias: Major causes include neonatal asphyxia, severe liver dz, drugs (e.g. valproic acid) , urea cycle disorders, organic acidurias, lactic acidoses, and dibasic amino acidurias.

  1. Rx: Arginine, sodium benzoate, phenylacetate, dialysis, and low-protein diet.

H. Leukodystrophies: Defects in myelin metabolism, usually lysosomal or peroxisomal, causing white matter dz and peripheral neuropathy. See below.

I. Lysosomal enzyme disorders: Glycoprotein degradation disorders, mucolipidoses, mucopolysaccharidoses, sphingolipidoses.

  1. Krabbe's leukodystrophy: (Globoid cell). Galactocerebrosidase deficiency. Onset in infancy, with irritability, hypertonia and opisthotonos, vision and hearing loss, seizures, ± peripheral neuropathy. Death in 2-3 yr.

  2. Metachromatic leukodystrophy: Arylsulfatase A deficiency. Infant to adult onset. May be spastic or flaccid. Severe peripheral neuropathy and CSF protein elevation. Also dementia, ataxia, optic atrophy.

  3. Others: Niemann-Pick, Gaucher's, or Tay-Sachs dz; GM1 gangliosidosis; Fabry's or Hurler's syndromes…

J. Peroxisomal disorders.

  1. Zellweger's syndrome: (Cerebrohepatorenal syndrome). Reduced or absent peroxisomes. Severe hypotonia, seizures, developmental delay, liver failure, and early death.

  2. Adrenoleukodystrophy: (ALD)

     a. Neonatal ALD and infantile Refsum's dz are milder variants of Zellweger's syndrome, above. N-ALD pts. benefit from docosahexaenoic acid.

     b. X-linked ALD Buildup of very long-chain fatty acids. Childhood-onset form starts with ADHD, progesses to seizures, dementia, ataxia, death. Adult-onset form (adrenomyeloneuropathy) causes progressive spastic paraparesis, sphincter trouble, and adrenal in-

sufficiency.
K. **Others:** e.g. metabolism of carbohydrate, glycoprotein, lipid, or purine; mucopolysaccharidoses, mucolipidoses; mitochondrial defects; endocrine defects.
  1. **Galactosemia:** Autosomal recessive defect in galactose-1-uridyltransferase.
     a. **H&P:** Usually normal at birth. First week: listlessness, jaundice, vomiting, diarrhea, no weight gain. Second week: hypotonia, cataracts, hepatosplenomegaly. Untreated infants get mental retardation and die of cirrhosis.
     b. **Tests:** Reducing substances in the urine; erythrocyte transferase activity.
     c. **Rx:** Lactose-free diet. Most treated infants have a normal IQ but visual-perceptual defects.
  2. **Hypothyroidism:**
     a. **H&P:** Post-term, macrosomic, jaundiced, large fontanelles, skin mottling, listless, big belly, umbilical hernia. By age 2 mo, hypotonic, grunting cry, wide-open sutures. Later, mental retardation, deafness, and spasticity.
     b. **Rx:** Thyroid replacement. Even with early rx, patients usually have learning and cerebellar disorders.
  3. **Mitochondrial disorders:** See p. 58.
  4. **Pyridoxine dependency:** Can cause neonatal seizures that respond only to pyridoxine.

MOVEMENT DISORDERS AND ATAXIA

A. **See also:** Adult movement disorders, p. 58.
B. **Ataxia:**
  1. **Acute or intermittent:** DDx includes
     a. **Cerebellitis:** Usually postviral, especially varicella and EBV. CSF shows mild lymphocytosis. Usually resolves completely.
     b. **Intoxication:** phenytoin, lead, alcohol, thallium,....
     c. **Occult neuroblastoma:** Usually with opsoclonus-myoclonus. Thought to be paraneoplastic.
     d. **Metabolic disorders:** Including maple syrup urine dz, Hartnup's dz, pyruvate decarboxylase deficiency, arginiosuccinic aciduria, hypothyroidism.
     e. **Paroxysmal disorders:** Seizure, migraine, benign positional vertigo, familial episodic ataxia.
     f. **Other:** Guillain-Barré syndrome, posterior fossa hemorrhage or stroke, MS.
  2. **Progressive ataxia:**
     a. **Congenital malformations:** Aplasias, Dandy-Walker or Chiari malformation.
     b. **Hereditary degeneration:**
        1) **Spinocerebellar ataxias:** Besides ataxia, there are often neuropathy, absent DTRs, weakness, and other organ system involvement, depending on the syndrome. This class includes SCA 1 through 7 (autosomal dominant), Machado-Joseph dz

(AKA SCA3) , Friedreich's syndrome (recessive), olivoponto-cerebellar atrophy. Genetic tests available for some.

  2) **Ataxia-telangiectasia syndrome:** A defect in DNA repair causing ataxia, telangiectasias, infections, and tumors.
  3) **Abetalipoproteinemia:** See p. 112.
  4) **Other:** Leukodystrophy, mitochondrial dz,....

  c. **Posterior fossa tumors:** See HA, vomiting (especially if early morning, not preceded by nausea), cranial nerve abnormalities, papilledema, meningismus.
  d. **Vitamin deficiencies:** e.g. E, B_{12}.

C. **Chorea:** Causes include Sydenham's dz, Wilson's dz, Huntington's dz, hyperthyroidism, vasculitis, basal ganglia tumors or strokes, estrogens, pregnancy, Hallervorden-Spatz dz.

  1. **Sydenham's chorea:** Poststreptococcal, in association with rheumatic fever. See also emotional lability and obsessive-compulsive behavior. Check antistreptolysin O titer. Pt. should get prophylactic penicillin until adulthood, as 1/3 will develop valvular dz.

  2. **Wilson's dz:** Autosomal recessive, copper builds up in liver and basal ganglia.
     a. **H&P:** Usually childhood onset. Cirrhosis, corneal Kayser-Fleischer rings, personality changes, and extrapyramidal sx including tremor, ataxia, dysarthria, and dystonia.
     b. **Tests:** Low serum ceruloplasmin, high urine copper, abnormal LFTs, subcortical and brainstem changes on CT or MRI.
     c. **Rx:** D-penicillamine 250-500 mg PO qid. Pyridoxine supplements. Side effects include transient decline of neurological function, allergic sensitivity, nephrotic syndrome, a lupus-like syndrome, low platelets, myasthenia, and Goodpasture's syndrome.

D. **Dystonia:** See also causes of chorea, above.
  1. **Drug effect:** e.g. from neuroleptic or antiemetic. See p. 60.
  2. **Idiopathic torsion dystonia:** (Dystonia musculorum deformans). Onset usually age 5-15, with action dystonia of one foot that then spreads. Often mistaken for hysteria. Often autosomal dominant in Ashkenazi families. Some response to high-dose anticholinergics.
  3. **Dopa-responsive dystonia:** Autosomal dominant, incomplete penetrance. Improves with sleep. Responds to low-dose levodopa.

E. **Tics:** Common in normal 6-9 year-olds. Tourette's syndrome is motor and vocal tics for more than 1 yr without interruption; often with ADHD, obsessive-compulsive disorder, echolalia, coprolalia, strong family history. For motor tics, consider clonazepam, clonidine or pimozide. For OCD, an SRI.

NEUROCUTANEOUS SYNDROMES

	Neurofibromatosis 1	Neurofibromatosis 2
Incidence	1/3000	1/30000
Onset of symptoms	Early childhood	Adolescence or adulthood
First symptoms	Café-au-lait spots, freckling	8th nerve problems
Acoustic schwannomas	Almost never bilateral	Hallmark of NF2
Typical tumors	Neurofibromas, astrocytomas	Schwannomas, meningiomas
Nontumor symptoms	Macrocephaly, low IQ, bone dz	Retinal dz, juvenile cataracts
Typical spine problems	Scoliosis, syringomyelia	Intradural tumors, syringomyelia
Screening MRIs?	Less useful	To catch 8th nerve tumors early
Risk of malignancy	Sarcoma, leukemia, pheochromo	No
Inheritance	Chromosome 17, dominant	Chromosome 22, dominant
Severity	Wide variation within a given family	Consistent within a given family

Table 29. Distinguishing NF-1 and NF-2.

A. Neurofibromatosis type I: (von Recklinghausen's dz)
  1. **H&P:** Family history of NF1; café-au-lait spots, neurofibromas, axillary or inguinal freckling, optic glioma, iris (Lisch) nodules, typical osseous lesion (thoracic scoliosis, anterolateral tibia bowing, pseudoarthrosis, sphenoid wing dysplasia).
  2. **Tests:** MRIs for symptoms; screening MRIs less useful.
  3. **Rx:** Surgery for symptomatic lesions.

B. Neurofibromatosis type II:
  1. **H&P:** Acoustic Schwannomas (usually bilateral, and before age 30), café-au-lait spots, posterior lens opacities, family history of NF2. No Lisch nodules; not associated with seizures, mental retardation, or macrocephaly.
  2. **Tests:** Screening MRI can detect acoustic tumors early.
  3. **Rx:** Resect acoustic Schwannomas before they cause deafness.

C. Tuberous sclerosis: Autosomal dominant gene on either chromosome 9 or 11, very variable expression. Many spontaneous mutations.
  1. **H&P:** Characteristic triad of seizures, retardation, and facial adenofibromas (misnamed adenoma sebaceum). See also hypomelanotic macules, shagreen patches (connective tissue hamartomas). Family history. Heart, pulmonary, and kidney tumors are often silent.
  2. **Tests:** MRI of head shows focal cortical dysplasias (tubers) and subependymal nodules. Renal, cardiac, and pulmonary screening.
  3. **Rx:** Steroids or vigabatrin for infantile spasms, anticonvulsants for seizures; resect intraventricular tumors causing hydrocephalus.

D. Sturge-Weber syndrome (encephalotrigeminal angiomatosis): Chromosome 3 defect, causes vascular port-wine nevus on face (usually in V1 distribution), contralateral hemiparesis and field cut, ipsilateral glaucoma, seizures, retardation.

E. von Hippel-Lindau dz: Dominant gene defect on chromosome 3. Not really a neurocutaneous disorder, but we had to stick it somewhere.
  1. **H&P:** Sx of hemangioblastomas, usually in posterior fossa, in 2nd to 4th decades. Also see retinal hemangiomas, renal cell carcinomas, pheochromocytomas.
  2. **Rx:** Early surgery for cerebral or spinal cord tumors, laser or cryosurgery for retinal tumors, frequent screening exams.

SEIZURES

A. See also: Adult seizures, p. 79, for classification, drug tables, etc.

B. Status epilepticus: <u>A medical emergency.</u> See p. 79.

C. H&P: Ask about birth history, maternal illnesses, precipitating factors, fever, skin color changes, movements, family history. Try to get parents to videotape an episode. Thorough skin and physical exam.

D. Tests:

1. **EEG:** Baseline rhythms change dramatically with age. Although interictal abnormalities may be present even if a seizure is not recorded, many pts. with epilepsy have normal EEGs. Sleep EEGs help – if necessary, give chloral hydrate 50 mg/kg PO, max 1000 mg. Consider continuous video-EEG monitoring.

2. **Labs:** Glucose, electrolytes, Ca, Mg, UA. In newborns and infants, consider ammonia, lactate, pH, metabolic screens.

3. **Head scans:** Intracranial ultrasound in newborns to rule out hemorrhage. CT in acute workups. MRI for structural detail.

E. Neonatal seizures:

1. **Sx during seizures:** Seizures in newborns are poorly organized and hard to tell from normal motor activity. Look for eye deviations, repetitive movements, tonic stiffening.

   a. Premature infants: Apnea and bradycardia may be the only sign.

   b. Intubated, chemically paralyzed infants: Sudden blood pressure changes may be the only sign.

2. **DDx:** Benign jitteriness, benign sleep myoclonus, nonconvulsive apnea, normal movement, opisthotonos.

3. **Causes of neonatal seizures:** The following time frames are not absolute.

   a. First 72 h of life: Hypoxic-ischemic encephalopathy, cerebral hemorrhage, bacterial meningitis, TORCH infection, cerebral dysgenesis, drug withdrawal, hyperammonemia, hypoglycemia, hypocalcemia, effect of local anesthetic, pyridoxine dependency. Rarely from inborn errors of metabolism.

   b. After 72 h: Cerebral hemorrhage, infection, hypocalcemia, inborn errors of metabolism, herpes simplex encephalitis, stroke, cerebral dysgenesis, kernicterus, benign familial neonatal seizures. Rarely from hypoxic injury.

4. **Rx of neonatal seizures:** Correct electrolyte abnormalities. If no hypoglycemia (< 30 mg/ml), give

   a. Phenobarbital: Load 15 mg/kg IV; may repeat to a total load of 40 mg/kg. Monitor SBP and breathing. Maintenance is 5 mg/kg qd, IV or PO, divided bid.

   b. Phenytoin: A second-line agent. Poorly absorbed PO in infants. Load 10 mg/kg IV x 2. Monitor cardiac rhythm. Maintenance 5 mg/kg qd.

F. Infantile seizures: (1 mo - 2 yr)

1. **DDx:** Apnea, migraine (can present as paroxysmal vertigo), paroxysmal dystonia, benign myoclonus, cyanotic syncope (usually triggered by anger or fear), pallid syncope (usually triggered by sudden pain). Both types of syncope can be associated with tonic/clonic movements.

2. **Simple febrile seizures:** Generalized, brief (< 15 min), single occur-

rences in a febrile illness.

    a. Relation to nonfebrile seizures: Febrile seizures are seen in 4% of children; only 2% of those will have epilepsy. Features that suggest epilepsy: neurodevelopmental abnormality, focal seizure, family history.

    b. Tests and rx: Unnecessary unless the seizure is focal, prolonged, or residual deficits persist. Children with frequent febrile seizures may receive prophylactic diazepam 0.33 mg/kg PO during a fever.

3. Nonfebrile seizures: Causes are similar in infants and children—see next section. The following are types of seizure that present between 1 mo and 2 yr.

    a. Infantile spasms: AKA West's syndrome.

        1) **H&P:** Onset is always before 1 yr. See brief myoclonic extensor or flexor spasms (salaam movements), sometimes mistaken for colic. "Symptomatic" spasms are associated with an abnormal baseline neurological exam; "cryptogenic" spasms with an initially normal infant.

        2) **EEG:** Usually shows hypsarrhythmia (chaotic, very high voltage slow waves and spikes) or burst-suppression pattern.

        3) **Rx:** ACTH, especially in cryptogenic cases (in which the ACTH toxicity is justified because the prognosis is slightly better). In symptomatic cases, where prognosis is poor, consider clonazepam.

    b. Myoclonic epilepsy: May be benign or severe.

        1) **H&P:** Brief seizures, no loss of consciousness, vary from head-nodding to sudden leg flexion and fall (with arms flung up and out). In severe myoclonic epilepsy, there is developmental delay and progressive ataxia and hyperreflexia.

        2) **EEG:** 3-Hz spike and wave in benign myoclonic epilepsy, > 3-Hz polyspike and wave in severe myoclonic epilepsy.

        3) **Rx:** Valproic acid 15 mg/kg qd divided bid. Watch closely for hepatotoxicity. Avoid carbamazepine, lamotrigine.

    c. Biotinidase deficiency

G. Childhood seizures:

1. DDx: Migraine, syncope, hyperventilation, narcolepsy-cataplexy, night terrors, startle dz (hyperekplexia), pseudoseizures, daydreaming.

2. Generalized tonic-clonic seizures: The most common type.

    a. H&P: See p. 81.

    b. Causes: Traumatic hypoxic, or ischemic brain injury, CNS infection, cerebral dysgenesis, metabolic abnormality, drug or toxin effect, drug withdrawal.

    c. Rx: No need to start anticonvulsants after a single seizure in an otherwise normal child. Phenobarbital (5 mg/kg qd), phenytoin (5 mg/kg qd—poorly absorbed in infants), and carbamazepine (load slowly to 15 mg/kg qd) are equally effective for recurrent seizures.

3. Simple partial seizures:

    a. H&P: Focal movement or dysfunction, often with subsequent secondary generalization.

    b. Causes: Benign centrotemporal or occipital epilepsy is the most common cause—see below. Any focal lesion, most often a neuronal migration disorder, mass, neurocysticercosis.

  c. Benign centrotemporal (rolandic) epilepsy: Genetic.

    1) **H&P:** Onset usually age 5-10; stop before age 14. Seizure usually during sleep, and wakes the child with mouth paresthesias and twitching for 1-2 min. Usually no LOC. Seizures sometimes spread to the arm or generalize.

    2) **EEG:** Interictal uni- or bilateral centrotemporal spikes, enhanced in sleep.

    3) **Rx:** Often unnecessary. Can try a single bedtime dose of phenobarbital.

  d. Benign occipital epilepsy: Probably genetic.

    1) **H&P:** Onset usually age 4-8; stop before age 12. Seizure usually has visual changes, often followed by migraine-like headache or nausea. Often induced by sleep-wake transition, photic stimulation, or video games.

    2) **EEG:** Interictal 2-Hz uni- or bilateral occipital spike-wave, inhibited by eye-opening.

    3) **Rx:** Standard anticonvulsants are usually successful.

4. Complex partial seizures: See p. 82.

5. Myoclonic seizures: See p. 118.

6. Absence seizures ("petit mal"):

  a. H&P: Onset 3-12 yr. Attacks last 5-10 sec, up to 100x qd. The child stares vacantly, sometimes with rhythmic eyelid movement. No aura or postictal confusion. Absence status can cause confusion. 50% of pts. with absence will also have at least one generalized seizure.

  b. Cause: Autosomal dominant trait with age-dependent penetrance.

  c. EEG: Bilateral synchronous 3-Hz spike-wave during the seizure. Can be triggered by hyperventilation.

  d. Rx: Ethosuximide, initial dose 20 mg/kg qd divided tid. Or valproic acid.

7. Landau-Kleffner syndrome:

  a. H&P: Onset age 2-11. Usually starts with selective word deafness or seizures (partial or generalized), followed by autistic personality changes.

  b. Cause: Unknown, except in rare cases of temporal lobe tumor. Hard to tell from autism, which may also have abnormal EEG.

  c. EEG: Multifocal parietal and temporal spikes.

  d. Rx: Anticonvulsants help the seizures but not aphasia. Early steroids may cause remission of aphasia and seizures.

8. Lennox-Gastaut syndrome:

  a. H&P: Seizures (atypical absence, atonic, and myoclonic), and mental retardation. Onset usually at age 1-5 yr. May follow infantile spasms.

  b. Causes: Usually from neurocutaneous disorder, peri- or postnatal brain injury.

  c. EEG: Slow (1-2.5 Hz) spike-wave complexes.

  d. Rx: Valproic acid, benzodiazepines, felbamate.

SOCIAL AND LANGUAGE DISORDERS

A. **Autism:** One of the pervasive developmental disorders.
   1. **H&P:** Usually normal early milestones, early language development followed by regression at age 1-2 yr. The classic triad is poor language, poor social interaction, and restricted or repetitive behavior and interests (abnormal imitative play, stereotyped movements such as whirling, rocking). Motor skills and memory may be normal.
   2. **Tests:** Audiology, EEG. Imaging usually not indicated.
   3. **Rx:** Behavioral therapy.
   4. **Syndromes with prominent autistic features:**
      a. **Fragile X syndrome:** Most common cause of mental retardation. See also dysmorphic facies, macro-orchidism after puberty, hyperactivity. 1/3 of female heterozygotes are also mildly retarded.
      b. **Angelman's syndrome:** ("Happy puppet" syndrome). Same 15q gene deletion as Prader-Willi syndrome, but of the maternal, not paternal chromosome. Infant feeding problems, severe retardation, autism, microcephaly, jerky puppetlike ataxia, paroxysmal laughter, protruding tongue. By contrast, Prader-Willi syndrome has severe floppiness at birth; dysmorphic, mental retardation, later hyperphagia, hypogonadism, Pickwickian syndrome.
      c. **Rett's syndrome:** Idiopathic, seen only in girls, in which autism is associated with progressive microcephaly, ataxia, breathing irregularities, seizures, scoliosis, spasticity, and dystonia.
      d. **Others:** Tuberous sclerosis, TORCH infections, phenylketonuria.

B. **Attention-deficit hyperactivity disorder:**
   1. **H&P:** Birth history, milestones. School performance—get detailed records. Are behavior problems limited to one domain? Staring spells? Family history of learning disability, stress, or substance abuse?
   2. **Tests:** Use DSM-IV criteria or Conners' motor overactivity scale.
   3. **Rx:** Methylphenidate 5 mg po q am, titrate up. Alternatives are dextroamphetamine and pemoline (watch LFTs on the latter). All can cause nausea, anorexia, insomnia, rebound hyperactivity. Tics may worsen.

C. **Dyslexia:**
   1. **H&P:** Family history of dyslexia or left-handedness. Selective difficulty reading and writing with intact visuospatial, mathematical, and memory abilities.
   2. **Rx:** Individualized educational intervention.

TUMORS

A. **See also adult sections:** Brain tumors, p. 90, and Spine tumors, p. 94.
B. **Infratentorial tumors:** The most common pediatric location. Pts. present with headache, ataxia, signs of high ICP or hydrocephalus, corticospinal and cranial nerve signs, head tilt, personality changes.
   1. **Brainstem gliomas:** Malignant. Usually no hydrocephalus until late. Peak incidence age 5-10 yr. Rx: XRT, dexamethasone.
   2. **Cerebellar astrocytoma:** Benign, usually cystic. Rx: surgery, usually no need for XRT.
   3. **Ependymoma:** Malignant, often along floor of 4th ventricle. Peak in-

cidence 0-4 yr. See early vomiting. Can seed spinal cord. Rx: surgery, XRT of head and spine.
   4. **Medulloblastoma:** Very malignant midline tumor, often in vermis. Peak incidence age 3-6 yr. Can seed spinal cord. Rx: surgery, XRT of head and spine, +/- chemotherapy.
C. **Supratentorial tumors:** Seizures and hemiparesis are common in supra- but not infratentorial tumors.
   1. **Craniopharyngiomas:** Suprasellar tumor, presents with signs of high ICP, pituitary dysfunction, or visual field deficits. Rx: surgery and XRT; prognosis relatively good.
   2. **Gliomas:** Rx of cerebral gliomas depends on the grade of the tumor. Rarely, children age 0-4 yrs present with weight loss despite a vora- cious appetite caused by a hypothalamic glioma.
   3. **Optic gliomas:** Present with poor vision, strabismus, exophthalmos, optic atrophy or papilledema. Surgery vs. XRT is controversial. When associated with neurofibromatosis, rx is sometimes conservative.
   4. **Primitive neuroectodermal tumors (PNETs):** Same pathology as medulloblastoma. Usually present in infancy. Rx: XRT of head and spine ± chemotherapy, survival poor.
D. **Intracranial metastases:** Rare in children, except from leukemia or lymphoma.
   1. **Leukemic infiltration of the meninges:** Pts. present with headache, papilledema, diplopia. To prevent this, methotrexate and XRT of head and spine are usually given during hematological remission; this can cause an encephalopathy.
   2. **Intracranial hemorrhage:** from low platelets; not seen in lymphoma.
   3. **CNS infection:** if peripheral white counts are low, CSF may not show lymphocytosis.

WEAKNESS

A. **See also:** Examination of infants, p. 101, Peripheral neuropathy, p. 72, Neuromuscular disorders, p. 62, Adult weakness, p. 99. The following fo- cuses on static or progressive weakness. Acute weakness suggests vascu- lar event or trauma. Subacute weakness suggests tumor, infection. If onset was prenatal, there is often arthrogryposis, dislocated hips.
B. **Hypertonic infants:** From CNS damage. Static hypertonia is usually cerebral palsy or a perinatal event; progressive hypertonia is usually a mass lesion or metabolic dz.
C. **Hypotonic infants:**
   1. **Upper motor neuron (CNS) causes:** See Developmental delay, p. 103. CNS hypotonia in infants usually has decreased tone with rela- tively preserved strength, in contrast to peripheral causes. CNS hypo- tonia progresses to hypertonia and spasticity.
   2. **Lower motor neuron, peripheral nerve, and muscle causes:** See below.
D. **Motor neuron dz:**
   1. **H&P:** Weakness, hypotonia, areflexia, fasciculations.
   2. **Tests:** CPK, NCS, EMG; consider genetic tests, e.g. for spinal mus- cular atrophy.

3. DDx:
  a. NCS normal:
  1) **Acute:** Polio, coxsackie virus, echoviruses.
  2) **Chronic:** Pure anterior horn cell sx suggest spinal muscular atrophy (SMA), e.g. acute infantile (Werdnig-Hoffman dz, AKA SMA-I) or late infantile (SMA-II). Additional lethargy suggests organic acidurias. Glycogen on muscle biopsy suggests Pompe's dz.

  b. NCS very slow: Do sural nerve biopsy; consider congenital hypomyelinating neuropathy, neuroaxonal dystrophy, infantile neuronal degeneration.

E. Spinal cord causes:
  1. **H&P:** Difficult or breech delivery, sensory level, sphincter disturbance.
  2. **Causes:** Trauma can present with hypotonia in newborns. Also consider tumor, hypoxic myelopathy.
  a. Atlantoaxial dislocation: From dislocation of C1-C2. Presents as acute or slowly progressive quadriplegia.
  b. Meningocele or spina bifida: See p. 105.
  c. Occult spinal dysraphism: AKA tethered cord syndrome, spina bifida occulta.
  1) **H&P:** Pts. present with back pain, bladder trouble, distal weakness or numbness, hemiatrophy, or scoliosis. Look for sacral dimple or lipoma, brisk leg reflexes.
  2) **Tests:** MRI shows a low-lying conus. A conus below L2-L3 is always abnormal in children over 5.
  3) **Rx:** Surgery (controversial).
  d. Syringomyelia: See Sensory loss, p. 83.

F. Peripheral weakness: Pts. are hyporeflexic with normal mental status.
  1. **Peripheral neuropathy:** Toxic, metabolic, traumatic (e.g. brachial plexus injuries, p. 75), Guillain-Barré syndrome, infectious.
  2. **Neuromuscular junction dz:** Myasthenia, botulism.
  3. **Myopathy :**
  a. H&P: Weakness usually worse proximally, reflexes not out of proportion to weakness. Look for muscle pain, steppage gait, waddle, trouble rising from floor, Gower's sign (walking hands up thighs to help straighten torso), atrophy, contractures, sometimes myotonia. Family history.
  b. Tests: CPK, EMG/NCS, muscle biopsy.
  c. DDx:
  1) **CPK markedly high:**
  a) **Inflammatory changes on biopsy:** Dermatomyositis or polymyositis. Gradual onset of weakness, malaise, muscle pain, fever, rash, edema. May cause GI ulcers or infarcts. Treat with high-dose steroids.
  b) **Muscle biopsy dystrophic:** Muscular dystrophy. Most common is Duchenne's, X-linked dystrophin deletion, with onset < age 5, proximal weakness, cardiac and GI involvement. Becker's is dystrophin alteration, onset > age 5, milder.

2) **CPK normal or mildly high:**
   a) **EMG and biopsy myopathic:**
      - **Maximal shoulder and hip weakness:** Endocrine, congenital, or metabolic myopathies, limb-girdle dystrophy.
      - **Other muscles involved early:** Dystrophies (fascioscapulohumeral, Emery-Dreyfuss, oculopharyngeal).
   b) **Myotonia present:** Myotonic dystrophy, myotonia congenita, paramyotonia.
   c) **Muscle weakness is intermittent:** Hypo- or hyperkalemic periodic paralysis, deficiency of phosphorylase, carnitine-palmital transferase, or phosphofructokinase.
   d) **Endocrine causes:** Myopathy from thyroid, parathyroid, or adrenal abnormalities (either hyper- or hypo-).
   d. **Rx:** Treat specific cause; close respiratory and cardiac follow-up, scoliosis screening.
G. **Genetic disorders causing isolated weakness:** Adrenoleukodystrophy, familial spastic paraplegia (a variant of spinocerebellar degeneration), spinomuscular atrophies, muscular dystrophies, metabolic myopathies.

DRUGS

ANGIOTENSIN-CONVERTING ENZYME INHIBITORS

A. **Indications:** To lower BP by decreased peripheral vascular resistance, with little change in cardiac output, HR, or glomerular filtration rate.
B. **Side effects:** Raises K. Dangerous in bilateral renal stenosis.

ADRENERGIC DRUGS

A. **See also:** ICU drips, p. 136.
B. α-receptor agents:
   1. **Endogenous ligands:** Epinephrine (E) and norepinephrine (NE) are approximately equipotent. Dopamine (DA) at high doses (> 10 μcg/kg/min) stimulates α–receptors (as well as β–receptors).
   2. **Location of receptors:** Mostly postganglionic sympathetic nervous system.
   3. α_1 **receptors:** Postsynaptic. Cause vasoconstriction, intestinal relaxation and sphincter constriction, increased heart contractile force, arrhythmias, pupillary dilation.
      a. **Selective agonists:** Phenylephrine, etc.
      b. **Selective antagonists:** Prazosin, etc. Peripherally acting.
   4. α_2 **receptors:** Presynaptic and nonneuronal. Causes platelet aggregation, lowers insulin secretion; lowers NE and acetylcholine release, some vasoconstriction.
      a. **Selective agonists:** Clonidine, etc. Centrally acting. Side effects include dry mouth, dizziness, constipation, low BP.
      b. **Selective antagonists:** Yohimbine, etc.
C. β receptor agents:
   1. **Non-selective agents:** Isoproterenol is an agonist; propanolol an antagonist, for both β_1 and β_2 receptors. DA at mid-range doses (> 2 μcg/kg/min) stimulates β–receptors much more than α–receptors.
   2. β_1 **receptors:** Cardioselective. Cause increased heart contractile force, HR, AV conduction; renin secretion. E and NE are approximately equipotent.
      a. **Selective agonists:** Dobutamine, etc.
      b. **Selective antagonists:** Metoprolol (low-dose), etc.
   3. β_2 **receptors:** Cause vasodilation and bronchodilation, intestinal relaxation. E is more potent than NE.
      a. **Selective agonists:** Albuterol, terbutaline.

ANALGESICS

A. **Acetaminophen:** 650 mg PO/PR q4h prn. Avoid in liver dz.
B. **TCAs:** See antidepressants, p. 130. For neuropathic pain.
C. **Na-channel blockers:** For neuropathic pain.
   1. **Carbamazepine:** See Anticonvulsants, p. 128.
   2. **Mexiletine:** IV lidocaine trial predicts effectiveness. Need to check

EKG first. Start mexiletine slowly to avoid GI side effects: 150 mg PO qd, then increase slowly to 300 tid; check level.
   3. **Gabapentin:** See Anticonvulsants, p. 128. Useful in reflex sympathetic dystrophy; migraine.
D. Nonsteroidal antiinflammatory drugs: For most types of pain; particularly bone pain and inflammation.
   1. **Dosing:** Ketorolac (Toradol) is the only NSAID that can be given IM; it is quick and effective, though expensive. When it is given PO, it has no more effect than ibuprofen. Ibuprofen PO may work more quickly PO than naproxen, although the latter requires less frequent dosing.
   2. **Side effects:** In one overall toxicity index, from safest to worst are salsalate, ibuprofen, naproxen, sulindac, piroxicam, fenoprofen, ketoprofen, meclofenamate, tolmectin, indomethacin.
      a. **CNS:** Analgesic rebound can cause headache when drug is discontinued after several days of use. High doses cause tinnitus. Ibuprofen has been associated with aseptic meningitis.
      b. **GI:** Nausea, bleeding. Consider checking stool guaiacs; GI prophylaxis, NSAIDS with reportedly fewer GI side effects (e.g. Trilisate), or giving in conjunction with misoprostol.
      c. **Antiplatelet:** Salsalate (Disalcid) may be less antiplatelet.
      d. **Renal:** Fluid retention, decreased glomerular filtration rate; can cause acute renal failure in high-catecholamine states; long-term use can cause interstitial nephritis.
E. Opiates: Good and underutilized for acute (e.g. post-op) pain. In chronic pain, do not confuse physical dependency (withdrawal sx when stopped suddenly) with addiction (escalating dose requirements without other evidence of dz progression).
   1. **Dosing:**
      a. **Longest-acting opiates:** MS contin, methadone, levorphanol, fentanyl patch. These are less likely to produce euphoria and dependence than short-acting opiates.
      b. **IV drip management:** When dose is increased, bolus with the difference, or it may take 12-24 h to reach new steady-state level.
   2. **Combination therapy:** Adding acetaminophen or an NSAID can decrease the need for opiates, even if NSAIDS were not effective as single agents.
   3. **Side effects:** Confusion, hypoventilation, constipation, addiction.
      a. **Overdose:**
         1) **H&P:** Dry mouth, dizziness, constipation, low BP. CNS and respiratory depression with small pupils.
         2) **Rx:** For respiratory depression, naloxone 2 mg IV; if only altered mental status, can try 0.4-0.8 mg. If pt. responds, give additional doses, preferably as continuous drip. Beware severe withdrawal sx in addicted patients.
      b. **Withdrawal:** From abrupt cessation of heavy prolonged use.
         1) **H&P:** muscle aches, lacrimation or rhinorrhea, pupillary dilation, sweating, diarrhea, yawning, fever, insomnia.
         2) **Rx:** Clonidine 0.15 mg PO bid, methadone 40 mg PO bid.
      c. **Analgesic rebound:** Can cause headache when opiate is discontinued, leading to a vicious cycle of dependence.

      d. **Constipation:** Put all pts. taking opiates on 2 Senekot tabs tid, Colace 100 mg tid, metoclopramide 10 mg tid. Lactulose is a good bail-out. Oral narcan can treat opiate-induced ileus: give 2-3 amp PO (or as enema) q 4h until bowel movement. It is expensive.

    4. Oxycodone: Usually available with acetaminophen (e.g. Percocet) or aspirin (e.g. Percodan). Short-acting.

    5. Morphine:

      a. **Histamine release:** Can cause itching. Consider fentanyl instead.

      b. **Nausea:** Consider hydromorphone instead (no 3-glucuronide metabolite).

    6. Meperidine (Demerol): Often given 25-100 mg IM, with 25 mg hydroxyzine (Vistaril), to prevent nausea. Metabolite buildup limits chronic use.

      a. **Contraindications:** Monoamine oxidase inhibitors (remember Libby Zion), seizures (metabolite lowers threshold); renal failure.

    7. Hydromorphone (Dilaudid): May be the strongest PO opiate—try 6 mg x 1, then 2-4 q4h PO/SQ. Very addictive.

    8. Fentanyl (Duragesic): Available as skin patch 2.5-10 mg q72h, for long-term pain management. Increase the dose very slowly; it takes days to reach a steady blood level.

Narcotic	IM/IV	PO	Duration (h)	Narcotic	IM/IV	PO	Duration (h)
Butorphanol	2	—	3-4	Methadone	10	20	4-6
Codeine	120	200	4-6	Morphine	10	60	3-7
Fentanyl	0.1	—	1-2	Nalbuphine	10	—	3-6
Hydrocodone	1.5	7.5	4-5	Oxycodone	15	30	4-6
Hydromorphone	1.5	7.5	4-5	Oxymorphone	1	6	3-6
Levorphanol	2	4	6-8	Pentazocine	30	150	2-3
Meperidine	75	300	2-4	Propoxyphene	—	130	4-6

Table 30. Equivalent narcotic doses.

ANESTHETICS

A. Thiopental: 50-mg test dose; then 100-200 mg. Onset 30 sec, lasts 5 min; consciousness returns in 30 min.

B. Propofol: Give 10-20 mg (= 1-2 ml) q10sec until induction.

C. Methohexital: More potent and shorter action than thiopental. Can induce seizures.

ANTIBIOTICS: See Infections, p. 176.

ANTICOAGULANTS

A. Contraindications to anticoagulation (relative): Large territory brain infarct, brain tumor, cerebral aneurysm, abdominal aortic aneurysm > 6 cm, fever/new heart murmur (?septic emboli), thrombocytopenia, SBP > 210, recent surgery or trauma, history of cerebral or severe GI bleed, cholesterol emboli.

    1. Complication prevention: Consider GI prophylaxis, checking frequent CBCs, stool guaiacs. Monitor relevant coagulation parameters (PT, PTT, or antifactor Xa).

B. Heparin: Goal PTT = 60-80, except as below. Watch for heparin-induced thrombocytopenia (see p. 156).

1. **For prophylaxis of DVT:** 5,000 U SQ bid.
2. **For rx of stroke, DVT, PE:**
   a. **Boluses:** Avoid them in stroke, unless there is brainstem ischemia or a fluctuating neuro exam. Use boluses in PE, MI. Typically 3,000-5,000 units.
   b. **Initial rate:** Typically 1000 U/h; give 600-800 U/h if pt. small, old, or frail; consider 1300-1500 for big young pts.
   c. **Sliding scale:** For bid PTT:

PTT	Dose correction
> 120	Stop heparin, recheck PTT "superstat" in 2 h.
100-119	Hold hep. x 2 h; decrease 200 U/h, recheck in 4 h.
90-99	Decrease 200 U/h
80-89	Decrease 100 U/h
60-79	No change
50-59	Increase 100 U/h
40-49	Increase 200 U/h
< 40	Bolus 3000, increase 200 U/h, recheck stat in 4 h.

Table 31. Insulin sliding scale.

3. **For rx of anticardiolipin Ab:** See Blood, p. 155.
C. Warfarin: (Coumadin). Goal PT/INR = 2-3 for stroke, A fib (unless under 65 with no risk factors), DVT, LV thrombus; 3-4.5 for mechanical valve. Typical load is 10 mg qd x 2 d, then 5 mg qd; decrease this for small or old pts. Overlap with heparin for at least 24 h of therapeutic PT, to prevent early paradoxical hypercoagulability. With an INR of 2-3, bleed rate per year is about 2%; 0.6% for cerebral bleed. Concomitant aspirin probably doubles the bleed rate.
1. **Drug interations:** (Partial list)
   a. **Drugs that decrease warfarin clearance, raise PT:** Acetaminophen, allopurinol, amiodarone, Bactrim, cimetidine, fluconazole, isoniazid, metronidazole, indomethacin, omeprazole, oral hypoglycemics, phenothiazines, quinidine, salicylates, TCAs.
   b. **Drugs that increase warfarin clearance, lower PT:** Barbiturates, oral contraceptives, rifampin.
D. Danaparoid: (Orgaran). A heparinoid. Use instead of IV heparin if patient has heparin-induced thrombocytopenia (see p. 156). Bolus 1250-200 U, then 400 U/h for 4 h, then 300 U/h for 4 h, then 150 U/h. After a few hours on 150 U/h, draw danaparoid level and antifactor Xa level; use these to adjust danaparoid rate.
E. Enoxaparin: (Lovenox). A low-molecular weight heparin fragment. Use instead of IV heparin to avoid IV and frequent PTT checks. Dose 1 mg/kg SQ bid. Check factor Xa levels.
F. Lepirudin: (Refludan). A leech-derived anticoagulant. Use instead of heparin in patients with heparin-induced thrombocytopenia (see p. 156). 0.4 mg/kg slow IV bolus, then 0.15 mg/kg/h. Adjust to keep PTT ratio (pt.'s PTT over median lab normal range) 1.5-2.5. If below target range, increase dose in increments of 20% every 4 h.
G. Reversing anticoagulation.

1. **Contraindications:** Prosthetic valve, basilar thrombosis, etc.
2. **Warfarin:** Vitamin K 1 mg IV/SQ to lower PT a little. 10 mg qd x 3 days normalizes it, but makes anticoagulation hard for the next week.
3. **Heparin:** Protamine 10-50 mg IV over 5 min. 1 mg reverses approximately 100 U of heparin.
4. **Others:** If active bleeding, consider fresh frozen plasma; DDAVP to boost platelets.

ANTICONVULSANTS

A. **See also:** Seizure classification, p. 81.
B. **Pregnancy and seizure drugs:** Put all young women on folate 1 mg qd. Carbamazepine decreases oral contraceptive levels. Anticonvulsants are teratogens, so taper drugs off before pregnancy, if possible. However, seizures can endanger the fetus too.
C. **Drug rash:** Stop likely cause immediately. Beware progression to Stevens-Johnson syndrome. Lamotrigine is most likely to cause a rash. Carbamazepine has some cross-sensitivity with phenytoin.
D. **Carbamazepine** (Tegretol):
   1. **Mechanism:** Stops high-frequency firing via Na channel.
   2. **Load:** Check CBC, LFTs, iron. Don't start if iron > 15 μg%. Autoinduces its metabolism, so load 200 mg qhs x 2 d, 200 bid x 2 d, then 200 tid, check levels after 3 d. Load slower as outpt. Check LFTs and CBC q mo.
   3. **Side effects:** Need to increase oral contraceptive dose. Check CBC, LFTs frequently at first. Watch for headache, nausea, diplopia, rash, low WBC, hepatitis, low Na.
   4. **Drug interactions:**
      a. **Carbamazepine lowers levels of:** Ethosuximide, tiagabine, topiramate, valproic acid, contraceptives (need to increase estrogen from 35 to 50 μg), steroids,warfarin, antipsychotics, cyclosporine.
      b. **Carbamazepine raises levels of:** Phenobarbital.
      c. **Carbamazepine levels raised by:** (Sometimes to <u>toxic</u> levels) Cimetidine, erythromycin, Ca channel blockers, propoxyphene, isoniazid, lamotrigine.
      d. **Lithium and carbamazepine:** Interact without raising level of either drug, but can cause confusion, ataxia, tremor, hyperreflexia.
      e. **To taper carbamazepine:** taper 200 mg qd q2wk.
E. **Ethosuximide:** (Zarontin): Starting dose is 20 mg/kg qd divided tid. For absence seizures. Acts on Ca channels in thalamus; also potentiates dopamine. Lowers carbamazepine levels.
F. **Fosphenytoin:** (Cerebyx). Dosed in mg phenytoin equivalents (PE). Status epilepticus load 1000 mg PE IV/IM, at < 150 mg/min. Maintenance 4-6 mg PE/kg IV/IM.
G. **Gabapentin:** (Neurontin). Load 300 mg PO qhs x 2 d, then 300 bid x 2 d, then 300 tid; max. 3600 mg qd. Enhances GABA synthesis, may inhibit Ca channels
H. **Lamotrigine:** (Lamictal). Levels raised significantly by valproic acid. Beware rash. Load slowly—at most 50 mg PO qhs x 2 wk, then 50 bid x 2 wk, then 150-250 bid. Slower if treating with valproic acid.

I. Phenobarbital: (Luminal). A barbiturate.

   1. **Contraindications:** Myasthenia, myxedema, porphyria, attention-deficit hyperactivity disorder, depression.
   2. **Side effects:** Sedation, nystagmus, ataxia.
   3. **Dose:** Typically 60 mg bid-tid qd, children 3-6 mg/kg qd.
   4. **Drug interactions:** Decreases levels of carbamazepine, lamotrigine, phenytoin (variable), tiagabine, valproic acid.
   5. **Overdose:** Similar to alcohol overdose. See ataxia, nystagmus, small reactive pupils, eventually respiratory depression and fixed and dilated pupils.
   6. **Withdrawal after heavy use:** Similar to delerium tremens. Timing varies with the half-life of the barbiturate used, but generally seizures, hallucinations, and fever begin on the second day of withdrawal.

J. Phenytoin: (Dilantin, DPH). Used frequently as first agent mostly because it can be loaded quickly. Try switching to something better-tolerated.

   1. **Contraindications:** Secondary or complete AV block, bradycardia, hypotension, low ejection fraction, pregnancy. All pts on phenytoin should take folate.
   2. **Side effects:** Sedation, nystagmus, ataxia, transient dystonias, and ophthalmoplegias, rash. Chronic use causes coarse features, gingival hyperplasia, ataxia, cerebellar atrophy.
   3. **Dose:** Start 300 mg PO qd; adjust per symptoms. Because of zero-order kinetics, at near-therapeutic doses a small dose change can cause large level changes. See Table 32.
   4. **Drug interactions:**
      a. **Phenytoin lowers levels of:** Carbamazepine, ethosuximide, primidone, topiramate, valproic acid, warfarin, steroids, cyclosporine, doxycycline, estrogen, furosemide, quinidine, rifampin, theophylline, vitamin D.

Present level (mg/dl)	Change to make (mg/d)
<6	100
6-8	50
>8	25

Table 32. Phenytoin dose adjustments for goal level of 10-20 mg/dl.

   a. **Phenytoin raises levels of:** Phenobarbital.
   b. **Phenytoin levels raised by:** Acute alcohol, Depakote, cimetidine and other H2 blockers, allopurinol, amiodarone, diazepam, estrogens, ethosuccimide, imipramine, isoniazid, phenothiazines, sulfonamides, salicylates, trazodone,....
   c. **Phenytoin levels lowered by:** Chronic alcohol, carbamazepine, sucralfate, Osmolyte, calcium antacids.
   5. **Mechanism of action:** Decreases posttetanic potentiation in Na channel.
   6. **Phenytoin levels:** In low albumin or renal failure, the plasma level should be adjusted. The adjusted level should be 10-20 μg/ml (or free level 1-2 μg/ml).
      a. **Low albumin:**
         Adjusted level = measured level / [(0.2 x albumin) + 0.1].
      b. **Renal failure:**

Adjusted level = measured level / [(0.1 x albumin) + 0.1].

7. **To raise subtherapeutic level:** Kinetics change from first-order to saturation near therapuetic dose, so can increase level by 100 mg qd if level < 8, but by no more than 50 if > 8.
   a. **IV dose** (mg/kg) = 0.7 x (desired - observed plasma conc.)
   b. **Oral dose** (mg/kg) = IV dose + 10%.
8. **To discontinue phenytoin:** Taper 100 mg qd every 2 wk.

K. **Valproic acid** (Depakote): Strictly, Depakote is divalproex. Valproate is Depakene; usually not as well tolerated. They act on chloride channel, GABA receptor.
   1. **Side effects:** Check LFTs. Nausea, weight gain, thin hair, teratogenicity, polycystic ovarian syndrome. Small increased risk of bleeding; pancreatitis, hepatitis.
   2. **Dose:** PO takes several weeks for effect. 5 days on each dose: 250 mg qd, 250 bid, 250 tid, 250-250-500. IV: 10-15 mg/kg qd divided tid.
   3. **Drug interactions:**
      a. **Divalproex lowers levels of:** Carbamazepine, phenytoin (total level, but free phenytoin levels increase), phenobarbital.
      b. **Divalproex raises levels of:** Ethosuximide, lamotrigine, (lower the dose from tid to bid), phenobarbital, primidone.
      c. **Divalproex levels raised by:** Aspirin.
   4. **To discontinue valproic acid:** Taper 250 mg qd q 2 wk.

ANTIDEPRESSANTS

A. **Serotonin reuptake inhibitors:** If you are patient, lower doses can provide significant relief with fewer side effects.
   1. **Serotonin syndrome:** A rare but potentially fatal syndrome characterized by confusion, hypertension, myoclonus, tremor, and autonomic instability. Lorazepam, serotonin-blockers, and nitroglycerin have been used to treat it.
   2. **Fluoxetine:** (Prozac). The most stimulating, least anticholinergic common SRI.
      a. **Dosing:** Start 10 mg q am, max. 80 qd—higher for obsessive-compulsive disorder, e.g. 100-120.
      b. **Side effects:** Anxiety, insomnia.
   3. **Sertraline:** (Zoloft). Intermediate in anticholinergic effect.
      a. **Dosing:** Start 50 mg qd; max. 200 qd.
      b. **Side effects:** GI.
   4. **Paroxetine:** (Paxil). The most sedating, most anticholinergic common SRI, but less so than the TCAs. May be the best antidepressant for bipolar dz.
      a. **Dosing:** Start 10 mg qhs; max. 50.
      b. **Side effects:** Nausea, sedation, dry mouth, urinary hesitancy, constipation, orthostasis.
B. **Tricyclic antidepressants:** (TCAs). Also good for neuropathic pain.
   1. **Side effects:** anticholinergic, antihistamine, α_1 adrenergic block, Na channel block, norepinephrine or serotonin reuptake block.
      a. **Anticholinergic effects:** See p. 134. Consider adding bethanechol to counteract these side effects.

1) **Highest:** Amitriptyline, imipramine. Avoid in older pts. or those with big prostates. Good for sleeplessness from pain.
2) **Lowest:** Desipramine, nortriptyline, venlafaxine.
   b. **α₁-adrenergic blocking effects:** Causes orthostatic hypotension, syncope. Consider EKG before prescribing TCAs in the elderly.
   c. **Antihistaminergic effects:** Sedating. High in doxepin.
   d. **Rx of overdose:** Symptomatic; gastric lavage, monitor ECG, keep blood pH > 7.45 with Na bicarbonate rapid IV injection to prevent arrhythmias. Diazepam usually helps CNS effects. Severe anticholinergic sx may require physostigmine 2 mg slowly IV, with repeat of 1-4 mg prn at 20-60 min intervals.
2. **Nortriptyline:** (Pamelor). Less anticholinergic than amitriptyline or imipramine.
   a. **Dosing:** Start 10-25 mg PO qhs x 1 wk; gradually increase to 75 qhs. Max. 125.
   b. **Side effects:** Dry mouth, constipation, urinary retention, sedation, orthostasis.
3. **Desipramine:** (Norpramin). A very activating TCA; least anticholinergic.
   a. **Dosing:** Start 25 mg PO q am x 3 d, then 50 x 1 wk, then 100. Max. 300.
   b. **Side effects:** Insomnia, anxiety, bundle-branch block.
4. **Amitriptyline:** (Elavil) Not well tolerated by patients; very anticholinergic.
   a. **Dosing:** Start 10-25 mg qhs x 1 wk; gradually load to 100. Max 150. Can be useful for insomnia at 10-25 mg qhs.
   b. **Side effects:** Sedation, dry mouth, urinary hesitancy, constipation, orthostasis.
5. **Venlafaxine:** (Effexor). May be as good as nortryptaline for neuropathic pain, and safer, because less anticholinergic. But side-effect = headache at high doses.

C. **Other antidepressants:**
1. **Buproprion:** (Wellbutrin). Well-tolerated in the elderly, and in manic-depression. Not sedating. Has some dopamine agonist effects.
   a. **Dosing:** 75 mg qd x 3 days, then 75 bid x 1 wk, then 150 bid. Max. 450 qd.
   b. **Side effects:** Lowers seizure threshold; avoid in alcoholics.

BENZODIAZEPINES

Generic name	Proprietary	Half-life (h)	PO dose (mg)	Liver metab?
Alprazolam	Xanax	12	0.25-0.5 tid	
Chlordiazepoxide	Librium	24	5-25 tid/qid	Yes
Diazepam	Valium	20-80	2-10 bid/qid	Yes
Lorazepam	Ativan	8-20	0.5-2 q6-8h	
Oxazepam	Serax	8	10-15 tid/qid	

Table 33. Benzodiazepines.

A. **Indications:** Anxiolysis, sedation, anticonvulsant, muscle spasms.
B. **Difficult or emergent sedation:** "5/2/1 IM": haloperidol 5 mg, loraze-

pam 2 mg, benztropine 1 mg. Diazepam is less well absorbed IM than lorazepam.

C. **Time course:** Diazepam has the shortest onset; oxazepam the shortest duration. Shorter acting drugs such as alprazolam can cause rebound anxiety.

D. **Mechanism:** Benzodiazepines are GABA-A receptor agonists.

E. **Side effects:** Respiratory depression, hypotension, mildly teratogenic during first trimester. Shorter acting ones are less sedating, cause more rebound and withdrawal. Never use them as analgesics; they can potentiate pain.

   1. **Withdrawal:** Can occur after prolonged use, so taper slowly. Sx similar to alcohol withdrawal; can be life threatening.
   2. **Overdose:** Can partially reverse effects with flumazenil. For benzodiazepine overdose, give flumazenil 0.2 mg (2 ml) IV over 30 sec, then 0.3 mg q min to effect, or until max. of 3 mg (10 doses). Half-life is 15 min - 2.5 h. Consider IV drip of 1 mg/h. Respiratory depression may <u>not</u> be reversed. Beware seizures.

F. **Comorbid dz:**

   1. **Liver failure:** In cirrhotics and the elderly, benzodiazepines metabolized in the liver—e.g. diazepam—can linger for weeks. Lorazepam or oxazepam, metabolized primarily in the kidney, are preferred. If pt. has hepatic encephalopathy, avoid benzodiazepines completely; use narcotics if sedation is required.
   2. **Kidney failure:** Use lorazepam or oxazepam (no active metabolites).
   3. **The elderly:** In general, oxazepam is better tolerated than lorazepam.

CALCIUM CHANNEL BLOCKERS

A. **Effects:**

   1. **Lower blood pressure:** Nifedipine > diltiazem > verapamil. They lower afterload because they dilate arteries more than veins.
   2. **Nodal blockade and negative inotropy:** Verapamil > diltiazem >>> nifedipine.
   3. **Migraine prophylaxis** (No controlled trials).

CHEMOTHERAPY
A. Antineoplastic agent side effects:

Drug	Heart	Liver	GI	Vasc.	Neuro.	Lung	Renal
Azathioprine		X	X				
Bleomycin			X			X	
Busulfan						X	
Carboplatin					X		
Carmustine (BCNU)		X	X		X	X	X
Cisplatin (CDDP)					& ototox		& hem. cyst.
Cyclophosphamide	X						
Cytarabine (Ara-C)			X		X		
Dacarbazine (DTIC)			X				
Doxorubicin (Adria.)	X		X	X			
Etoposide (VP-16)					X		
Fluorouracil (5-FU)			X				
Ifosfamide	X	X					hem. cyst.
Methotrexate		X	X			X	X
Mitomycin C			X	X		X	
Taxol	X				X		
Vinblastine				X	X		
Vincristine				X	X		

Table 34. Antineoplastic agent side effects.

B. Neurological complications of cancer: Metastases; encephalopathy (metabolic, drug, or radiation-induced), paraneoplastic syndromes, CNS infection, infarct or bleed, myopathy (steroid-induced, cachectic), myositis, myasthenic syndromes.

C. Neurological side effects of chemotherapy by class:
  1. **Alkylating agents:**
     a. **Nitrogen mustards:** Cyclophosphamide, melphalan, chlorambucil. Neurological side effects rare.
     b. **Nitrosureas:** Lomustine (CCNU), carmustine (BCNU). BCNU causes leukoencephalopathy at high doses. CCNU causes blindness in combination with cranial irradiation.
  2. **Antimetabolites:**
     a. **Folate analogs:** Methotrexate.
        1) **Acute transient chemical meningitis:** 4-6 h after intrathecal dose, in ~10% of pts.
        2) **Transient encephalopathy:** 7-10 d after third or fourth intrathecal dose, in ~4% of pts.
        3) **Transverse myelopathy:** After intrathecal dose, uncommon, paraplegia often permanent.
        4) **Leukoencephalopathy:** Weeks or months after brain XRT plus intrathecal or high-dose IV methotrexate.
     b. **Pyrimidine analogs:** 5-Fluorouracil, cytarabine. Occasional transient cerebellar dysfunction. Cytarabine sometimes causes neuropathy.
     c. **Purine analogs:** Azathioprine, fludarabine. Avoid allopurinol.
  3. **Natural products:**
     a. **Vinca alkaloids:** Vincristine, vinblastine. Especially vincristine: peripheral nerve dysfunction, usually hours to days after dose, usu-

ally reversible. Worse if liver dz. See autonomic dysfunction and
ileus (metoclopramide can help), decreased reflexes, toe and finger
paresthesias, weak foot and wrist.

   b. Abx: Daunorubicin, doxorubicin, bleomycin, mitomycin. Neurological effects rare.
   c. Other: Etoposide, L-asparaginase. L-asparaginase causes encephalopathy, usually transient, in ~15% of pts; also stroke or
   cerebral bleed in ~2% (drug-induced coagulopathy).
 4. Hormonal agents: Tamoxifen, flutamide, leuprolide. Neurological
    side effects rare.
 5. Other: Cisplatin, hydroxyurea, procarbazine, mitotane, aminoglu-
    tethimide. Cisplatin (but not carboplatin) causes hearing loss, dose-
    dependent large-fiber sensory neuropathy; sx can progress even after
    drug stopped. Sometimes seizures, confusion (but r/o Mg and Ca
    wasting). Procarbazine can cause encephalopathy and peripheral neu-
    ropathy.

CHOLINERGIC DRUGS

A. Location of receptors: Preganglionic sympathetic nervous system (SNS)
   + parasympathetic nervous system (PSNS), postganglionic PSNS, postganglionic SNS for sweating and vasodilation.
B. Acetylcholinesterase inhibitors: Inhibit acetylcholine breakdown, e.g.
   neostigmine (does not penetrate CNS well), physostigmine, (does).
C. Muscarinic receptors: Postganglionic. Cause small pupils, high heart
   rate, secretions, bronchospasm, and bladder tone. Agonists include
   bethanechol, glycopyrrolate. Antagonists include benztropine, tri-
   hexyphenidyl, scopolamine, atropine.
D. Nicotinic receptors: Found in preganglionic ANS (where hex-
   amethonium is an antagonist), and at the neuromuscular junction (where
   curare is an antagonist).
E. Anticholinergic toxicity: Mad as a hatter (delirium). Dry as a bone (dry
   mouth, anhidrosis). Blind as a bat (blurred vision). Plugged as a pig (stool
   and urinary retention). Hot as a hare (fever). Fast as a fibrillation
   (tachycardia).

DIGOXIN

A. Elimination: Renal. However, digoxin can't be dialyzed off.
B. Drug interactions: Cut digoxin dose in half when you start verapamil,
   quinidine, or amiodarone; check frequent levels.
C. Overdose: (Note digoxin level must be drawn > 6 h after dose).
   1. Signs: Vomiting, diarrhea, diplopia, yellow-haloed vision, confusion,
      low KCl. Long PR interval, heart block, junctional tachycardia, V
      tach, and V fib. Bidirectional V tach is pathognomonic for dig. toxic
      ity.
   2. Rx: Cardiac monitor; stop digoxin, replete KCl, Mg, and Ca; lido-
      caine for V tach/V fib. If heart block, pace. Digibind only if serious ar-
      rhythmia.

DIURETICS

A. Acetazolamide: (Diamox). A carbonic anhydrase inhibitor that raises extracellular carbon dioxide and decreases CSF formation. It is used in pseudotumor cerebri and sometimes as an adjunct anticonvulsant. Side effects: rash, agranulocytosis, paresthesias. Follow CBC, electrolytes.
B. Furosemide: (Lasix). A loop diuretic. 10-40 mg IV bolus; 20-80 mg PO qd-bid. Side effects: low BP, low K, ototoxicity.
C. Mannitol: Osmotic diuretic used to lower intracranial or intraocular pressure. 25% mannitol is 1375 mOsm/L. Cleared renally in about 3 h, but ICP effect lasts 3-8 h. See p. 54.

DOPAMINERGIC DRUGS

A. Dopamine: used to increase heart rate, contractility, and SBP. Can cause arrhythmias. See ICU drips, p.136.
B. Dopamine (DA) receptors:
  1. D1 receptors: Cause vasodilation.
  2. D2 receptors: Inhibit sympathetic transmission, inhibit prolactin release, cause vomiting.
  3. D3, 4, 5 receptors: Less well characterized; limbic more than motor effects.
C. Agonists: Used mostly for Parkinson's dz.
  1. Levodopa: A precursor to dopamine. Given with carbidopa, which blocks peripheral, but not central, levodopa use. Start 25/100 (carbidopa/levodopa) qd, bring to tid. If necessary, give up to total 1000 mg qd of levodopa, dosing q2-4h. Carbidopa dose should be > 75 mg; > 125 may cause nausea. Take Sinemet > 30 min before or >60 min after meals.
    a. Side effects: N/V, low BP, confusion, dyskinesias, hallucinations.
  2. Receptor agonists: Side effects are like levodopa, but agonists are less likely to cause dyskinesias, more likely to cause confusion.
    a. D3 agonists: e.g. pramipexole (Mirapex). Start 0.125 mg tid, max 1.5 mg tid. Or pergolide (Permax). Start 0.05 mg qd, max 1.5 mg tid.
    b. D2 agonists: e.g. bromocriptine (Parlodel), ropinirole (Requip).
  3. Inhibitors of DA metabolism:
    a. Monoamine oxidase inhibitors:
      1) **MAO-B inhibitors:** e.g. selegiline (Eldepryl). They slow dopamine degradation. Start 2.5 mg bid, to 5 bid.
        a) **Side effects:** N/V. Avoid opiates, TCAs, and SRIs (can cause hyperthermia, rigidity, autonomic instability).
      2) **Nonspecific MAOIs:** Used as antidepressants. <u>Many</u> dietary and drug contraindications, notably meperidine, SRIs.
    b. Carboxy-o-methyltransferase (COMT) inhibitors: e.g. tolcapone (associated with fulminant liver failure). For end-stage Parkinson's.
  4. Amantidine: DA agonist, mechanism unclear, also anticholinergic and antiviral. Used for Parkinson's dz, fatigue in MS.
    a. Side effects: Rare confusion, depression, edema.

D. Antagonists: Neuroleptics, e.g. haloperidol. Used for sedation, psychosis, vomiting. Extrapyramidal side effects are proportional to D2 binding. Clozapine requires close monitoring for agranulocytosis.

Generic name	Trade name	Sedation, dizziness	Rigidity	Receptor	First dose (mg)
Traditional neuroleptics					
haloperidol	Haldol	+/-	++++	D2, high	0.5-5
perphenazine	Trilafon	++	++	D2, med	2-10
thioridazine	Mellaril	++++	+/-	D2, low	10-100
Atypical neuroleptics					
clozapine	Clozaril	++++	-	5-HT > D2	25
risperidone	Risperdal	+/-	+/-	5-HT > D2	0.5-2
olanzepine	Zyprexa	+	-	5-HT $\cong$ D2	5-10
quetiapine	Seroquel	+	-	α > D2	25

Table 35. Neuroleptics.

E. Neuroleptic-induced movement disorders:
   1. Neuroleptic malignant syndrome (NMS): <u>An emergency</u>. Caused by a sudden release of calcium from sarcoplasmic reticulum as idiopathic response to a neuroleptic, or to withdrawal of antiparkinsonian drug.
      a. H&P: Recent drugs. See tachycardia, then acidosis, tachypnea, arrhythmias, muscle stiffness, and fever.
      b. DDx of NMS: Malignant hyperthermia, drug interactions with MAOIs, central anticholinergic syndromes, catatonia,....
      c. Tests: ABG, electrolytes, CBC, CPK, EKG.
      d. Rx of NMS:
         1) **Transfer to ICU, maintain ventilation.**
         2) **Surface and core cooling.**
         3) **Dantrolene:** Start 1 mg/kg IV, repeat prn to 10 mg/kg qd. Watch for hepatotoxicity, CHF.
         4) **Bromocriptine:** Start 2.5-10 mg IV/pNGT q4-6h.
   2. Acute dystonia: Within a few days of drug initiation. See Dystonia, p. 60, for rx.
   3. Akathisia: See above.
   4. Subacute parkinsonian sx: Days to weeks after drug initiation. Treat by switching to an atypical neuroleptic; add an anticholinergic drug (No indication for prophylactic use).
      a. Benztropine 0.5-4.0 mg bid.
      b. Trihexyphenidyl 1-5 mg bid-tid.
   5. Tardive dyskinesia: Choreoathetosis, dystonia, orobuccal dyskinesia as late (> 1 yr) response to chronic neuroleptic use. Switch to an atypical neuroleptic. Avoid anticholinergics. Consider tetrabenazine, reserpine.

ICU DRIPS

A. See also: Adrenergic drugs, p. 124; Dopaminergic drugs, p. 135.
B. Access: Most require central line.
C. Dobutamine: To treat heart failure. Increases cardiac output while decreases SVR, so BP often doesn't change. Doesn't increase capillary

wedge pressure as much as DA does.

D. Dopamine (DA): To treat low BP, bradycardia, e.g. in RV infarct, or oliguric renal failure (controversial). Low doses can be given by peripheral IV.

   1. **Side effects:** Arrhythmia, tachycardia (especially if pt. is hypovolemic).
   2. **Low-dose effects:** 0.5-3 µg/kg/min. Causes renal dilation, Na excretion, via DA receptors.
   3. **Medium-dose effects:** 5-10 µg/kg/min. Causes positive inotropy, via β–receptors.
   4. **High-dose effects:** >15 µg/kg/min. Causes vasoconstriction, via α–receptors. High doses sometimes dilate and even fix pupils.

E. Epinephrine: To treat anaphylaxis; to help circulation in cardiac codes.

F. Lidocaine: To decrease ectopy. Dangerous in bradycardia or AV block.

G. Nitroglycerine (TNG, NTG): To treat cardiac ischemia, coronary or esophageal spasm, CHF if BP not low. Low doses can be given by peripheral IV. It causes venous greater than arterial dilation. May reduce cardiac output. Unlike nitroprusside, it does not cause cerebral steal.

H. Nitroprusside (NTP): To treat high BP in stroke, hyptertensive crisis, aortic dissection. It causes arterial dilation and venodilation equally. Avoid in ischemic brain; it may cause cerebral steal by dilating peripheral vessels. Low doses can be given by peripheral IV. After 3 d of use, check thiocyanate levels daily.

I. Norepinephrine (Levophed): To treat low BP in sepsis. β_1 and α–receptor effects. Inotropic at 1-2 µg/min; then vasoconstriction and venoconstriction.

J. Phenylephrine (Neosynephrine): To treat low BP in stroke; second-line agent for septic shock. Pure α–receptor effects, no β (vasoconstricts without inotropy), so increases afterload without inotropic support.

Category	Target	Dose Per Kg	Average Dose	Toxicity
Pressors				
dopamine (Intropin)	D1, D2	0.5–2 µg/kg/min	50-150 µg/min	↑ HR, arrhythmia, big pupils
	β, D	2–10 µg/kg/min	200-500 µg/min	HTN
	α, β, D	>10 µg/kg/min	500-1000 µg/min	
norepinephrine (Levophed)	α1, α2 β1>β2		1–16 µg/min	vasospasm, acute renal failure
phenylephrine (Neosynephrine)	α1		10-300 µg/min	vasospasm, acute renal failure
dobutamine (Dobutrex)	β1	2–20 µg/kg/min	100-1000 µg/min	arrhythmia, initial ↓ SVR
epinephrine (Adrenalin)	α1, α2 β1, β2		0.25-4 µg/min	vasospasm, MI, arrhythmia
isoproterenol (Isuprel)	β1, β2		0.1-20 µg/min	arrhythmia, MI, hypotension
amrinone (Inocor)	PDE-III inhibitor	0.75 mg/kg then 5-15 µg/kg/min	40 mg over 3 min then 250-900 µg/min	HR ↑, platelets ↓, hypotension

Category	Target	Dose Per Kg	Average Dose	Toxicity
Cardiac				
lidocaine	Na chan-nel	1 mg/kg then 1-4 mg/min	bolus 70-100 mg then 1-4 mg/min	confusion, seizures, arrhythmia
procainamide	Na, K channels	15 mg/kg @ 50 mg/min, 1-4 mg/min	1 gram over 20 min then 1-4 mg/min	hypotension, long QT interval
bretylium	K channel	5 mg/kg then 1-4 mg/min	350-700 mg then 1-4 mg/min	hypotension, ar-rhythmia
amiodarone	K channel	150-300 mg then 0.4-0.8 mg/kg/h	150-300 mg over 5 min then 3-6 mg/h	hypotension, ar-rhythmia
nitroglycerin	smooth muscle		10-1000 µg/min	BP ↓, hypoxia, methemoglobin
nitroprusside (Nipride)	direct vascular	0.1–10 µg/kg/min	5-800 µg/min	thiocyanate toxicity
esmolol (Brevibloc)	β1>β2 blocker	500 µg/kg then 25–300 µg/kg/min	20-30 mg over 1 min then 2-12 mg/min	CHF, hypotension
enalapril (Vasotec)	ACE-I	0.625–1.25 mg over 5 min then 0.625–5 mg q6h		K ↑, BP ↓, acute renal failure
hydralazine (Apresoline)	direct vasodilator	5-20 mg q3 min up to 400 mg then 5-20 mg q6h		angina, hypotension
labetalol (Normodyne)	α1, β1, β2 blocker	2.5–10 mg then 10–120 mg/h or 2.5-10 mg q15 min		negative inotrope, BP ↓
verapamil (Calan)	Ca chan-nel	2.5–15 mg then 5-20 mg/h		AV block, BP ↓
diltiazem (Cardizem)	Ca chan-nel	0.25 mg/kg over 2 min, reload 0.35 mg/kg q15 min prn, then 10-15 mg/h		AV block, BP ↓
nicardipine (Cardene)	Ca chan-nel	5 mg/h, titrate by 2.5 mg/h q5-15 min then ↓ rate by 1-7.5 mg/h when goal BP reached		BP ↓

Table 36. ICU drips.

IMMUNOSUPPRESSANTS

A. Side effects: Immunosuppressants of all types increase the risk of opportunistic infections and malignancy, especially lymphoma.

B. Azathioprine: An antimetabolite. Coadministration with allopurinol will increase its toxicity. Marrow and liver side effects.

C. Corticosteroids:

    1. Indications: For brain tumors, multiple sclerosis, other inflammation….

    2. Side effects:

        a. Endocrine: Glucose intolerance, adrenal insufficiency after withdrawal of steroids, hirsutism, growth retardation.

        b. Electrolytes: Na and water retention, low K. Give KCl supplements.

        c. Musculoskeletal: Osteoporosis, myopathy. Give calcium + vitamin D between steroid courses (risk of kidney stones when given together.

        d. Connective tissue: Centripetal obesity, striae, poor wound healing.

        e. Immune: Increased infections, decreased allergic reactions, increased WBC count.

    f. GI: Ulcers. Give ulcer prophylaxis.

    g. CNS: Insomnia, mania, psychosis. Lithium 300 mg qd can help.

  3. Adrenal insufficiency after withdrawal: Taper steroids slowly to avoid insufficiency.

D. Cytoxan: An alkylating agent. See Chemotherapy, p. 133.

E. Cyclosporine: Inhibits T cells. Major side effects are renal. Some patients get cyclosporine headaches that are dose dependent; may benefit from propranolol or gabapentin.

F. FK506: (Tacrolimus) Inhibits T cells. Major side effects are renal. Some patients get FK-506 encephalopathy, with MRI showing white-matter dz. This is sometimes reversible with stopping FK506.

G. Interferon: Cytokines with immunosuppressive and antiviral effects. β-interferon is used in MS. Side effects include a flu-like syndrome, marrow suppression, and rare confusion or seizures.

H. Methotrexate: An antimetabolite; see Chemotherapy, p. 133.

MUSCLE RELAXANTS

A. See also: Benzodiazepines, p. 131.

B. Baclofen: A GABA-B agonist. For spasticity, back pain, trigeminal neuralgia.

  1. Dosing: Start 5-10 mg PO bid, to 10-30 tid.

  2. Side effects: Sedation, weakness, nausea, depression. If stopped suddenly after several weeks of heavy use, can trigger seizures.

C. Dantrolene: A direct muscle relaxant.

  1. Dosing: See p. 136 for dosing in neuroleptic malignant syndrome. For spasticity, start 25 mg PO qd, up to 400 mg qd divided bid/qid.

  2. Side effects: Hepatotoxicity, CHF, sedation.

D. Tizanidine: (Zanaflex) α_2-adrenergic agonist, used for spasticity.

  1. Dosing: Varies widely across pts, from 2 to 39 mg PO qd; must titrate over 2-4 wk, as it takes about a week to reach max. effect.

  2. Side effects: Sedation, weakness (less than baclofen), dry mouth.

E. Quinine: Frequently used for leg cramps, although not FDA approved for this.

  1. Dosing: try 300 mg PO qhs.

  2. Side effects: Cinchonism with overdose. Hemolysis with G-6PD deficiency.

PARALYTICS

A. Pupils are spared: Large pupils in a patient given paralytics is usually evidence of anxiety from inadequate sedation.

B. Succinylcholine: 1-1.5 mg/kg IV bolus (typically 3.5-5 ml/70 kg of 20 mg/ml solution), onset 60-90 sec, lasts 3-10 min. Infusion 2.5-15 mg/min. A depolarizing blocker that can cause autonomic stimulation and raise ICP. Blunt this by pretreating with pancuronium (nondepolarizing) 1 mg IV, 5 min before succinylcholine.

C. Vecuronium: 0.07-0.1 mg/kg IV bolus (typically 8-10 mg/70 kg), 2-3 min onset, lasts 15-30 min. Nondepolarizing.

IMAGING

ANATOMY

A. Opposite of neuropathological conventions: Besides the obvious fact that radiological images are presented with anatomical left on the right side of the picture, remember that the brainstem on a horizontal MRI is upside down compared with textbook images of the brainstem in coronal section.

B. Sections:
   1. **Axial** (horizontal): Parallel to ground if patient were standing. The standard section. In the spine, gives a cross-section.
   2. **Coronal:** Not in plane with a crown, but a coronet, or one of those preppy headband things. Good for pituitary, skull-base, orbital, and hippocampal lesions.
   3. **Sagittal:** In plane with the interhemispheric fissure. In the spine, gives a longitudinal section.

C. Landmarks:
   1. **Ventricles and cisterns:** In horizontal section, the ventricles look like a face, with lateral ventricles for eyes, third ventricle for a nose, and a mouth whose sides are the perimesencephalic (or ambient) cisterns and whose base is the quadrigeminal cistern below the colliculi. It should be smiling—flattening of the quadrigeminal cistern suggests herniation.
   2. **Central sulcus:** In horizontal section, it is most easily seen in upper-most sections, where it has a characteristic sickle shape. The superior frontal sulcus, running parallel to the falx, terminates in the pre-central sulcus; the central sulcus is just posterior.
   3. **Orbit:** There is proptosis if more than half the eyeball sticks out past the line between the zygoma and the nose.

D. Pediatric neuroimaging: See p. 103 for patterns of myelination.

ANGIOGRAPHY

A. Indications: Cerebral bleeds when you suspect aneurysm or AVM. Cerebrovascular stenosis that is equivocal on ultrasound, MRA or CT angiography. Vasculitis. To characterize blood flow near a tumor before surgery.

B. Interventional angiography: Includes coiling of aneurysms, intra-arterial thrombolysis, glue embolization of AVMs, partial embolization of tumors or epistaxis.

C. Orders: NPO after midnight, IV fluids, pre-op labs (CBC, PT, PTT, electrolytes).

D. Consent: Risk of complication $\cong$ 4%; permanent $\cong$ 1%, death $\cong$ 0.6% Higher risk with interventional procedure, tight stenosis, or h/o migraine.

E. Sheath pull: Normally done by the neurointerventional team at the end of the angiogram, but it is sometimes left in for longer. Percutaneous closure devices may be used. Must be done surgically in anticoagulated pts.

F. Anatomy: see also Vascular territories, p. 22.

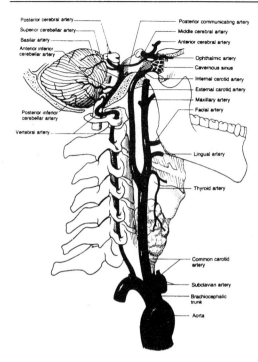

Figure 13. Carotid artery anatomy.(From Duus P. *Topical Diagnosis in Neurology*. New York: Thieme, 1983:415, with permission.)

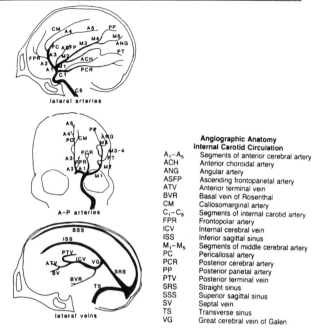

	Anglographic Anatomy Internal Carotid Circulation	
A_1–A_5	Segments of anterior cerebral artery
ACH	Anterior choroidal artery
ANG	Angular artery
ASFP	Ascending frontoparietal artery
ATV	Anterior terminal vein
BVR	Basal vein of Rosenthal
CM	Callosomarginal artery
C_1–C_5	Segments of internal carotid artery
FPR	Frontopolar artery
ICV	Internal cerebral vein
ISS	Inferior sagittal sinus
M_1–M_5	Segments of middle cerebral artery
PC	Pericallosal artery
PCR	Posterior cerebral artery
PP	Posterior parietal artery
PTV	Posterior terminal vein
SRS	Straight sinus
SSS	Superior sagittal sinus
SV	Septal vein
TS	Transverse sinus
VG	Great cerebral vein of Galen

Figure 14. The carotid circulation. (From Lerner AJ. *The Little Black Book of Neurology*, 3rd ed. St. Louis: CVMosby, 1995:20, with permission.)

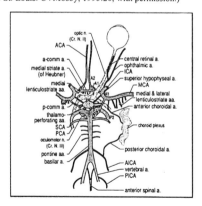

Figure 15. The circle of Willis. (From Greenberg MS. *Handbook of Neurosurgery*, 3rd ed. Greenberg Graphics, 1994:109, with permission.)

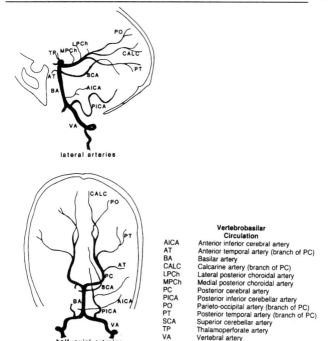

Figure 16 The vertebrobasilar circulation. (From Lerner AJ. *The Little Black Book of Neurology*, 3rd ed. St. Louis: CVMosby, 1995:21, with permission.)

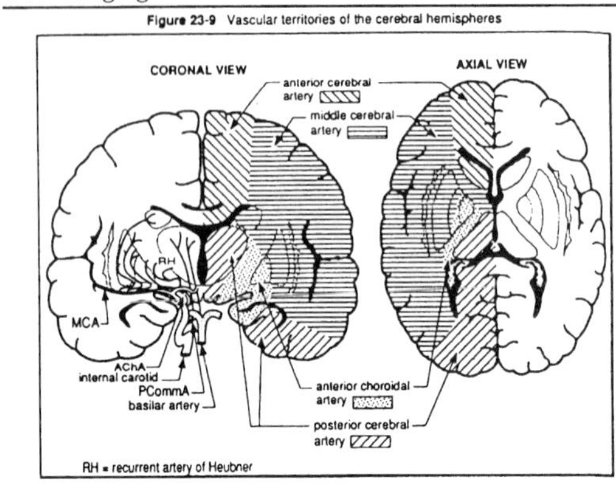

Figure 23-9 Vascular territories of the cerebral hemispheres

Figure 17. Cerebrovascular territories. (From Greenberg MS. *Handbook of Neurosurgery*, 3rd ed. Greenberg Graphics, 1994, with permission.)

COMPUTERIZED TOMOGRAPHY (CT)

A. Indications for noncontrast study: Bleeds, old cerebral strokes, hydrocephalus, edema, skull fractures, intracranial air, calcifications, metal in head. Good for acute or unstable pt., or pt. who can't have MRI.

B. Indications for contrast: Large tumor or abscess, extensive meningeal inflammation.

C. Indications for CT myelogram: Spinal cord lesion in pt. with multiple back surgeries, metal implants causing artifact, or who can't get an MRI. Doesn't show lateral or foraminal herniations.

D. Indications for CT angiogram (CTA): Decisions about thrombolysis in pts. with acute stroke. Vascular lesion in pt. who can't get an MRI. Specify the area of interest. Remember, CTA is not a dynamic study—a vessel may fill but have very sluggish flow.

E. What CT is bad for: Posterior fossa and brainstem (much artifact), small lesions, subacute blood (isodense with brain).

F. Relative contraindications:
   1. **Noncontrast:** Limit use in first trimester pregnancy. Unstable pts. should not be sent to the scanner unmonitored.
   2. **Contrast:** Renal failure; creatinine should be < 2.0. Previous contrast reaction. Contrast can sometimes trigger flash pulmonary edema. See Allergy, p. 154, for prevention and rx of contrast allergies.

G. DDx by CT appearance: Bone > clotted blood > liquid blood > subacute (~2 wk) blood ≅ brain tissue > CSF > water > fat.
   1. **See also:** DDx by MRI appearance, p. 150, for the DDx of ring-enhancing lesions, etc.
   2. **Hyperdense (bright) lesions:** Recent blood, metastases (often), meningioma, calcification, bone.
      a. **Calcifications:** Seen in oligodendroglioma, toxoplasmosis, neurocysticercosis, meningioma, Fahr's syndrome, AVM, calcified an-

eurysms, neonatal infections.

3. **Hypodense (dark) lesions:** Infarct (after 12-36 h), primary brain tumors (often), inflammation, old blood, edema, posttraumatic changes, fat, cysts, air.

4. **Ventriculomegaly:** Obstruction, atrophy, normal pressure hydrocephalus.

H. CT of specific lesions:

1. **Infarct:**

   a. **Acute:** Infarcts are often hard to see for 12-24 h. Large strokes may show early loss of gray-white differentiation, or of sulcal defintion.

   b. **Subacute:** Hypodensity in the distribution of a single vascular territory. Look for edema, mass effect, or hemorrhagic conversion. Some tiny lacunar strokes may never be visible by CT. Strokes 2-4 wk old may have ring- enhancement with contrast.

   c. **Chronic:** Hypodensity, often with tissue loss that may cause sulcal or ventricular widening.

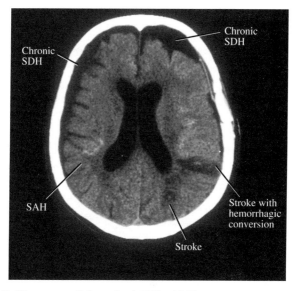

Figure 18. CT appearance of infarcts, chronic SDH, and SAH.

2. **CT signs of intracranial hemorrhage:** See also p. 50.

   a. **Epidural hematoma:** High-density biconvex (lens-shaped) area next to skull. Does not cross sutures. Often with skull fracture.

    b. Subdural hematoma (SDH): High or heterogeneous density, crescentic area next to skull. Crosses sutures, but not the midline. Look for edema, shift, cortical flattening, associated fracture or scalp bruise. Subacute SDH may be isodense; see only obliteration of sulci and midline shift. There may be no shift if SDH is bilateral.

    c. Subarachnoid hemorrhage (SAH): 95% sensitive if done within 48 h. Serpentine density in sulci, fissures, and basal cisterns, often dissecting into ventricles. Look for associated fracture or scalp bruise, hydrocephalus, hematoma that may need evacuation. Often can predict aneurysm location. If suspicion of SAH but negative CT, should do an LP.

    d. Intracerebral hemorrhage (ICH): Hyperdense blood, often surrounded by edema. Location is guide to cause.

       1) Contusion: Often frontal or temporal pole often with contracoup contusion in opposite occipital lobe. Petechial hyperdensity associated with hypodensity, skull fracture or scalp bruise.

       2) Hypertensive bleed: Usually in basal ganglia, brainstem, cerebellum, or white matter.

       3) Amyloid bleed: Usually at gray-white junction. Get an MRI with iron susceptibility sequence to see additional occult lesions that help confirm the diagnosis.

  3. Intracranial pressure: Look for sulcal effacement, midline shift, distortion of nearby structures by mass. <u>The absence of the fourth ventricle is a neurological emergency.</u> The fourth ventricle should be visible even in the presence of significant beam-hardening artifact.

    a. Hydrocephalus: Frontal horns and third ventricles balloon ("Mickey Mouse" ventricles), periventricular low density from transependymal absorption of CSF. In children, plain skull films may show splayed sutures.

       1) Obstructive hydrocephalus: Obstruction gives large lateral ventricles with effacement of sulci. Third or fourth ventricle may look closed. There is usually a visible compressing lesion.

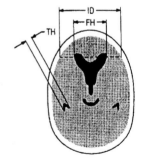

       2) Communicating hydrocephalus: All ventricles and the cerebral aqueduct should be large. In hydrocephalus from atrophy, sulci are widened, whereas in hydrocephalus from CSF malabsorption (e.g. after SAH), they may be narrowed.

Figure 19 . Ventricular parameters in hydrocephalus. (From Greenberg MS. *Handbook of Neurosurgery*, 3rd ed. Greenberg Graphics, 1994:224, with permission.)

       3) Ratios that suggest hy-

drocephalus: Temporal horns ≥ 2 mm for both temporal horns (see Figure 19) and *either*
   a) **Sulci and fissures are invisible,** *or*
   b) **FH/ID > 0.5:** where FH = largest width of frontal horns and ID is internal diameter of brain at this level.

4) **Chronic hydrocephalus:** Erosion of the sella turcica with third ventricle herniating downward. Atrophy of corpus callosum on sagittal MRI. In children, macrocephaly.

b. **CT signs of herniation:**

   1) **Subfalcine:** Cingulate gyrus is displaced across the midline under the falx. May have enlargement of contralateral ventricle.

   2) **Central transtentorial:** Obliteration of the perimesencephalic and quadrigeminal cisterns, sometimes with PCA territory infarcts and small Duret hemorrhages in the brainstem.

   3) **Uncal transtentorial:** Early: flattening of the normal pentagonal shape of the suprasellar cistern (see "Ventricles and cisterns," p. 140). Later: brainstem displacement, compression of contralateral cerebral peduncle, sometimes contralateral hydrocephalus. Finally: obliteration of parasellar and interpeduncular cisterns.

   4) **Tonsillar:** Cerebellar tonsils in foramen magnum, best seen on sagittal section. Tonsils should be less than 5 mm beneath base of occipital-clival line.

   5) **Upward cerebellar:** Vermis is above tentorium; may compress quadrigeminal cistern, sylvian aqueduct and cause hydrocephalus.

4. **CT signs of head trauma:**

   a. **Contusion:** Predominantly gray-matter hypodensity. See intraparenchymal blood, usually with little mass effect, usually in poles of cerebral hemisphere, next to bone.

   b. **Shear injury (diffuse axonal injury):** Seen especially after deceleration injury. Little change in CT; in severe cases may see petechial hemorrhages in white matter and brainstem. Best evaluated by MRI.

   c. **Skull fracture:** May be complicated by epidural hemorrhage or CSF leak. Fluid in a sinus or mastoid suggests an occult fracture.

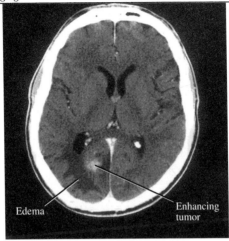

Edema

Enhancing
tumor

Figure 20. CT with contrast, of tumor and surrounding edema.

    5. CT signs of tumor: Sensitive enough for most cortical tumors large
enough to be symptomatic, but small metastases, posterior fossa tumors, and some isodense gliomas will require MRI.
        a. Mass: With contrast, most tumors are bright or ring-enhancing.
Without, they may be dark or isodense, sometimes seen only by
disortion of adjacent structures. Look always for L-R asymmetries.
        b. Associated findings: Look for dark edema surrounding the tissue,
midline shift, hydrocephalus, herniation, blood, infarcts. In infants,
because there is no gray-white differentiation, it is easy to miss
small amounts of edema.
        c. DDx: Inflammation and enhancing subacute infarcts may look like
tumors.

MAGNETIC RESONANCE IMAGING (MRI)

A. Indications: Posterior fossa or small supratentorial lesions, distinguishing between new and old strokes, white matter dz, nonacute seizure
workup, AVMs,....
    1. For gadolinium: Good for hyperperfused structures, e.g. inflamma-
tion, tumors.
    2. For MR angiogram: For head or neck arterial stenosis. Gives more
anatomical information than ultrasound, but tends to overestimate severe stenoses. You can also request an MR venogram to rule out venous sinus thrombosis.
    3. What MRI is bad for: Imaging blood (especially acute); bone, cal-
cium. MRI is almost never the choice for acute problems, except in
certain stroke protocols.
B. Contraindications:
    1. Implants: <u>Cardiac pacemakers.</u> Other metallic foreign bodies or im-

plants in head. Ferromagnetic aneurysm clips, e.g. Drake, Heifetz, mayfield, Scoville. However, modern clips are usually MRI compatible, including Olivecrona, Sugita, McFadden, and Yasargil.

2. **Unstable pts:** Medical monitoring in the scanner is often hard. Pts. with claustrophobia or back pain will benefit from premedication with benzodiazepines or opiates, respectively.

3. **Size:** Pts. over 300 lbs. may not fit. Doubt colleagues who tell you that the veterinary school nearby has a horse scanner that will take large humans. At least in Boston, this is an urban myth.

4. **Contrast:** Rarely a problem. Gadolinium is safe for pts. with renal failure or CT contrast allergies.

C. **Sequences:** TE is echo time, TR is repetition time.

1. **T1-weighted:** Good for disorders of CSF circulation, contusions, subacute blood. TE < 50, TR < 1000.

   a. **Bright:** Fat, gadolinium, methemoglobin (subacute hemorrhage, see p. 150), proteinaceous substances, melanotic tumors, mineralization.

   b. **Dark:** CSF, bone, edema, deoxyhemoglobin in intact RBCs. Most pathology is dark, but a notable exception is subacute hemorrhage.

   c. **Contrast studies:** Almost always done with T1 weighting. The contrast is gadolinium and does not contain iodine. Look at cerebral veins or nasal mucosae to see if scan is gadolinium enhanced.

2. **T2-weighted:** Good for infarcts, inflammation, tumors. TE > 80, TR > 2000. More contrast with longer TE.

   a. **Bright:** CSF, liquids, edema. Most pathology is bright.

   b. **Dark:** Solids, calcium, hemosiderin, deoxy- and methemoglobin in intact RBCs, ferritin, mucinous metastases.

3. **Proton density, AKA spin density:** Fat and water are gray, most pathology is bright. TE < 50, TR > 2000.

4. **Fluid-attenuated inversion recovery (FLAIR):** Like T2, but CSF is dark. Edema and gliosis are bright. TE > 80, TR > 10,000. Good for small white matter lesions, and those near CSF.

5. **Diffusion-weighted image (DWI):** Good for acute infarcts (see p. 151). T2-bright lesions may "shine through," mimicking an infarct. Low resolution. Bright artifact at air-bone interfaces.

6. **Susceptibility sequence:** Good for imaging hemorrhage (even after reabsorption), calcifications. Metals, e.g. the iron deposits of microhemorrhages, create dark areas larger than the lesion's actual extent.

7. **MR angiogram:** Good for vessels. Does not use contrast—a gradient echo sequence makes blood bright. The standard sequence selects for blood traveling at arterial speed, but you can also request an MR venogram, which shows vessels with slower blood flow. Phase contrast MRA or MRV shows flow velocity and direction.

8. **Short tau inversion recovery (STIR) image:** Causes fat to drop out; good for spine and orbit.

9. **MR spectroscopy:** Experimental; good for tumors and metabolic disorders.

10. **Functional MRI:** Good for preoperative localization of cortical areas. Shows focal changes in blood flow that correlate with focal brain activity.

D. DDx by MRI appearance:

1. **Ring-enhancing lesions:** "MAGIC DR." Metastases, Abscess/aneurysm, Glioblastoma, Inflammation (resolving stroke, infection), Contusion (resolving), Demyelination (active), Radiation necrosis.

2. **Gray-white junction lesions:** Metastases, septic emboli, thrombosis, vasculitis.

3. **Periventricular lesions:** MS, hypertensive microvascular dz, toxoplasmosis, CNS lymphoma, CMV, lacunar infarcts, glioma.

4. **Cerebello-pontine angle lesions:** "SAME." Schwannoma, Arachnoid cyst, Meningioma, Epidermoid.

5. **Basal ganglia lesions:** Bleed, stroke, carbon monoxide, lead, methanol, Creutzfeldt-Jacob dz, TORCH infection.

E. MRI of specific lesions:

1. **Abscess:** T2 hyperintense ring of edema and hypointense capsule, enhances with gadolinium. Bright on DWI.

2. **Amyloid angiopathy:** Iron susceptibility sequence shows dark regions at sites of old bleeds.

3. **Arteriovenous malformations:** Serpiginous hyper- and hypodensities on T2 MRI; tangle of vessels on MRA.

4. **Brainstem lesion:** Request thin cuts through the brainstem.

5. **Carotid or vertebral artery lesion:**
   a. **Stenosis:** MRA of neck and head. Few false negatives, but frequent false positives.
   b. **Dissection:** Order T1 neck axials with fat saturation and MRA. 90% sensitive.

6. **Chiasm/optic nerve/middle fossa problem:** Order gadolinium and fat suppression (STIR sequence), with coronal cuts through orbit and middle fossa.

7. **Edema:** Bright T2 and FLAIR.

8. **Hemorrhage dating:** Complicated. CT is better for fresh blood. Dating depends on the oxidation state of the hemoglobin. The clot oxidizes from the outside, in, giving a ring appearance at some stages.
   a. **T1 appearance:** Gray → white →black (mnemonic = George Washington Bridge).
   b. **T2 appearance:** Black → white → black (mnemonic = oreo cookie).

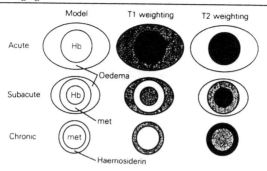

Figure 21. Variation with age of ICH appearance on MRI. (From Berlit P. *Memorix Neurology.* Chapman and Hall, 1996, with permission.)

9. **Infarct:**
   a. **Acute and subacute infarcts:** Diffusion-weighted image (DWI) is bright within 30 min and for 2 wk poststroke. After 4-12 h, see bright T2, bright FLAIR, bright proton density, dark T1. There may be edema or punctate hemorrhage associated with subacute infarcts.
   b. **Chronic infarcts:** Similar to subacute infarcts except that they are not bright on DWI and may show tissue loss or cavitation rather than edema or hemorrhagic conversion.
10. **Multiple sclerosis:** T2-bright white matter lesions, usually periventricular, with long axis perpendicular to ventricles (Dawson's fingers). Acute plaques may ring-enhance.
11. **Tumor, brain:** T1 and T2 density will vary with tumor type, presence of hemorrhage. etc. Look for hydrocephalus, shift, necrosis, enhancement, edema. See also Brain tumors, p. 91.
    a. **Gray-white junction:** Mass suggests metastasis.
    b. **Hemorrhagic mass:** Suggests GBM, metastasis.
    c. **Calcification:** Suggests oligodendroglioma, meningioma, vascular malformation.
    d. **Lymphoma:** Homogeneous enhancement, often subcortical, little edema. In AIDS, may ring enhance and look like toxoplasmosis.
    e. **Meningioma:** Extraaxial, usually dark on T2, enhances uniformly (lightbulb sign).
    f. **Pituitary tumor:** Specify MRI with thin cuts thru sella. To see microadenoma, scan must be done within 5 min of gadolinium (normal pituitary enhances immediately, but microadenoma takes about 30 min).
    g. **Post-op scans:** Should be done within 48 h, to see residual tumor before inflammation begins. Post-op pituitary scan may not be helpful.

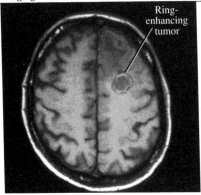

Ring-
enhancing
tumor

Figure 22. MRI with gadolinium showing ring-enhancing mass.

12. **Tumor, spinal cord:** Multiple lesions are common, so request longitudinal scout of entire spine. Consider gadolinium.
   a. **Intramedullary:** Astrocytoma, ependymoma.
   b. **Intradural:** Nerve sheath tumor, meningioma, lymphoma.
   c. **Extradural:** Metastases; bone tumor.
13. **Vertebral disc herniation:** On T2 images, compressed discs are darker; they bulge into CSF (bright) and sometimes spinal cord (grey). Axial cuts show nerve root impingement best.

ULTRASOUND

A. **Carotid and/or vertebral duplex:** (AKA carotid noninvasives, CNIs). For stenoses in neck vessels. Uses B-mode and pulsed Doppler imaging.
B. **Transcranial Doppler:** (AKA TCDs). For stenoses in intracranial vessels. Specify anterior and/or posterior circulation TCDs when ordering. Add TCDs to CNIs if there is > 60% carotid stenosis on CNI. Can also help identify vasospasm, AVMs, absence of cerebral blood flow in brain death.
C. **Neonatal brain ultrasound:** For bleeds, periventricular leukomalacia, and congenital malformations, in pt. with an open fontanelle.

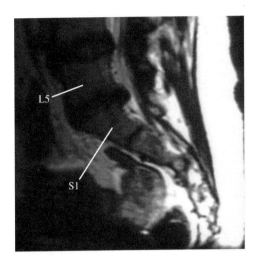

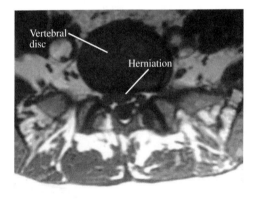

Figure 23. The parasagittal and axial T2-weighted MRI images show a right paracentral disc herniation toward the proximal right S1 nerve root.

MEDICINE

ALLERGY

A. Rx of anaphylaxis:
1. **Maintain airway:** Consider intubation.
2. **Diphenhydramine:** IM 50 mg.
3. **Epinephrine:**
   a. **Standard:** 0.3-0.5 ml of 1:1000 SQ (= 0.3-0.5 mg) q15-20 min.
   b. **Elderly or in shock:** Dilute 0.1 ml of 1:1000 in 10 ml NS; then give it IV over 5-10 min.
   c. **Stridor:** Racemic epinephrine nebulizer.
4. **Steroids:** e.g. dexamethasone 10-40 mg IV.

B. Premedication to prevent iodinated contrast reaction: Use nonionic contrast. Give prednisone 30 mg PO 12 h and 2 h before; diphenhydramine 50 mg PO 2 h before.

BLOOD

A. Anemia
1. **Neurological complications of anemia:** Headache, lightheadedness. Sickle cell anemia can cause strokes, seizures, or extramedullary hematopoesis in the meninges that mimics masses.
2. **H&P:** H/o ulcers, liver dz, easy bleeding, ecchymoses, stool guaiac, jaundice, adenopathy.
3. **Tests:** CBC, BUN/Cr. Consider reticulocyte count, smear for morphology, iron, TIBC, ferritin, bilirubin, endoscopy or abdominal CT, SIEP, Hb electrophoresis, haptoglobin, Coombs test, bone marrow biopsy.
4. **Causes of anemia:**
   a. **Acute:** Bleeding.
   b. **Subacute:** Bleeding, hemolysis.
   c. **Chronic:**
      1) **Low reticulocyte count** (decreased production):
         a) **Low MCV** (microcytic):
            - **Iron deficiency:** Fe and ferritin down, TIBC up. Usually from bleeding. Consider endoscopy. Treat with ferrous sulfate 325 mg tid if Fe/TIBC ratio is < 20%.
            - **Anemia of chronic dz:** Fe down, ferritin up (only if ESR is up), TIBC down.
            - **Others:** Thalassemia, sideroblastic anemia.
         b) **Normal MCV** (normocytic): Bone marrow failure, either secondary (kidney, liver, or other chronic dz) or primary.
         c) **High MCV** (macrocytic): B_{12} or folate deficiency, drug-induced, liver dz, hypothyroidism.
      2) **High reticulocyte count** (increased production): Bleeding, hemolysis (antibody-mediated, traumatic, toxic, intrinsic cell defect).

5. **Rx of acute or severe anemia:** : Blood bank sample, type and cross 2 U, guaiac stools, consider transfusion, gastric lavage. For active bleeding, place two 14-ga IVs, start saline, consider medicine or GI consult.

   a. **Bleed on anticoagulants:** Reverse anticoagulation. See p. 127.

   b. **Transfusions:** 1 U packed red blood cells (PRBC) should raise Hct 3 pts.

      1) **Typical transfusion order:** Transfuse 2u PRBC over 4 h each; premed before each unit with acetaminophen 650 mg PO and diphenhydramine 50 mg PO.

      2) **If danger of CHF,** or if pt. <u>severely</u> anemic, premedicate with 20 mg furosemide IV before each unit.

      3) **If danger of transfusion reaction,** e.g. if pt. has received many transfusions, request leukopoor or washed RBCs.

      4) **If pt. has suppressed marrow,** use irradiated RBCs.

   c. **Transfusion reaction:** Call blood bank.

      1) **H&P:** Sudden fever (most common), sweating, hives, wheezing, tachycardia, hypotension.

      2) **Rx:** Stop blood product. Diphenhydramine and acetaminophen if mild. If severe, add hydrocortisone 50-100 mg IV. If hemolysis, maintain diuresis with IV fluids and furosemide.

B. Coagulopathy:

1. **Neurological complications of coagulopathy:** Stroke, hemorrhage, headache, lightheadedness, neuropathy (especially femoral, from retroperitoneal bleed). Paraprotein can cause neuropathy.

2. **H&P:** Look for hematomas, signs of liver or autoimmune dz, tumor.

3. **Tests:** Check platelets, PT, PTT, fibrinogen, D-dimer, protein C and S (can't be tested on warfarin), antithrombin III (can't be tested on heparin), anticardiolipin and antiphospholipid antibodies. Consider Russell viper venom test, ESR, RF, ANA.

4. **Causes of abnormal coagulation:**

   a. **Long PTT:** Heparin, anticardiolipin Ab, lupus anticoagulant, intrinsic pathway defect, hemophilia.

   b. **Long PT:** Warfarin, vitamin K deficiency, liver dz, DIC, extrinsic pathway defect.

   c. **Long PT and PTT:** Very high levels of warfarin; common pathway defect, some lupus anticoagulant.

   d. **Other hypercoagulable states:** DIC, tumors, pancreatitis, vasculitis, oral contraceptives, smoking, DM, nephrotic syndrome, anticardiolipin Ab, lupus anticoagulant, homocysteinuria, thrombocytosis, leukostasis. Deficiency of protein C, activated protein C, protein S, or antithrombin III.

5. **Anticoagulants:** See p. 126.

6. **Antibody-mediated coagulation disorders.** Consider hematology consult. Often an antibody will be present without abnormal clotting or bleeding.

   a. **Lupus anticoagulant (antiphospholipid Ab):** Despite its name, it more commonly causes thrombosis than bleeding. Clots are usually venous. PTT is high in 50%. Rare pts. also have high PT; they are at risk for bleeding.

    b. Anticardiolipin Ab: Causes either arterial or venous clots, and pts. who have had one or the other tend to continue to have that kind. PTT is usually normal.

    c. Rx: A thrombotic event is an indication for warfarin or heparin therapy. See Anticoagulants, p. 126, for contraindications. With heparin, if PTT is already falsely elevated, the PTT goal is approximately 2x the pt.'s baseline. It is more accurate to follow heparin level (goal 0.2-0.4), or thrombin time (TT, goal 2-3 x control).

C. Disseminated intravascular coagulation: Often post-op, or from sepsis. Platelets and fibrinogen are low, PT, PTT, and D-dimer are high.

    1. Rx of DIC: Treat underlying cause; if necessary, replace with fresh frozen plasma, platelets, cryoprecipitate, blood. Heparin is usually not indicated, unless there is evidence of thrombosis (e.g. stroke, digit ischemia, or oliguria despite good SBP) or in some malignancies. Never give heparin if there has been head trauma.

D. Erythrocyte sedimentation rate: Nonspecific, but useful to rule out temporal arteritis, cancer, chronic infection.

    1. Normal for women = (age)/2 + 10.

    2. Normal for men = (age)/2.

E. Eosinophilia: Mnemonic for causes is <u>NAACP</u>—<u>N</u>eoplasm, <u>A</u>ddison's dz, <u>A</u>llergy, <u>C</u>ollagen vascular dz, <u>P</u>arasites.

F. Heparin-induced thrombocytopenia:

    1. H&P: Platelets fall while patient is receiving heparin.

    2. Dx: Blood assay for heparin-induced thrombocytopenia (HIT test).

    3. Rx: Change heparin to danaparoid or hirudin (see anticoagulants, p. 126).

G. Platelet disorders:

    1. Neurological complications of platelet problems: See Coagulopathy, p. 155.

    2. H&P: NSAID or heparin use? Look for petechiae, mucous membrane bleeding.

    3. Tests: Consider bleeding time, von Willebrand's factor test.

    4. Contraindications: Platelets < 100, no surgery. Platelets < 50, no minor procedures. Platelets < 20, bleed from minor trauma. Platelets < 10, spontaneous bleeding (except in idiopathic thrombocytopenic purpura, where remaining platelets are hyperactive).

    5. Causes: DIC, drug reaction, e.g. heparin-induced thrombocytopenia, idiopathic thrombocytopenic purpura, thrombotic thrombocytopenic purpura, SLE.

    6. Rx: Think twice about platelet transfusion (not in DIC or thrombotic thrombocytopenic purpura, where pt. may be hypercoagulable. Not helpful if cause is autoimmune or drug-induced). Try Amicar, DDAVP. Autoimmune problem may be helped with steroids, IgG, pheresis.

H. Thrombotic thrombocytopenic purpura:

    1. H&P: Low platelets, microangiopathic hemolytic anemia, altered mental status (often with seizures); fever, renal problems.

    2. Rx: Pheresis.

EPIDEMIOLOGY

A. Sensitivity: The probability that a test will be positive if the condition it tests for is present: (true positives)/(true positives + false negatives).
B. Specificity: The probability that a test will be negative if the condition it tests for is absent: (true negatives)/(true negatives + false positives).
C. Bayes' theorem: The likelihood of a patient's having a condition given a positive test result (i.e. the positive predictive value, PV^+) depends on the frequency (f) of the condition in the population:
$$PV^+ = (f)(sensitivity)/[(f)(sensitivity) + (1-f)(1-specificity)]$$

ELECTROLYTES

A. Tests:
   1. Arterial blood gases and serum electrolytes:
      a. pH < 7.38 implies acidosis; pH > 7.42 implies alkalosis.
         1) **Respiratory vs. metabolic pH changes:** If pH change is purely respiratory, for every change in pCO_2 of 10 torr, there should be 0.8 pH unit change. Greater or less than this implies superimposed metabolic process.
      b. Bicarb < 24 implies metabolic acidosis.
         1) **Anion gap** = Na - Cl - bicarb. Normal is < 12 ± 4.
            a) **Correction for low albumin:** Normal anion gap = 2x(albumin) + 4.
            b) **Correction for alkalosis:** A pH > 7.5 causes a high anion gap just by uncovering negative sites on albumin.
         2) **Is there respiratory compensation for the metabolic acidosis?** If 1.5x(bicarb) + (8 ± 2) > pCO_2, then there is. But if it is < p CO_2, then there is a superimposed respiratory acidosis.
      c. Bicarb > 24 implies metabolic alkalosis. Look at pCO_2 (below) to see if there is a concurrent respiratory alkalosis.
      d. pCO_2: If pCO_2 < 40, there is an added primary respiratory alkalosis. If pCO_2 > 50, there is a primary respiratory acidosis.
         1) **Acute:** If for every 10 mm Hg pCO_2 above (or below) normal, the pH is below (above) normal by 0.08.
         2) **Chronic:** If for every 10 mm Hg pCO_2 above (or below) normal, the pH is below (above) normal by 0.03.
   2. Venous blood gases: Can be used to estimate arterial blood gases.
      a. Arterial bicarb = venous bicarb + 2.
      b. Arterial pCO_2 = venous pCO_2 - 6.
      c. Arterial pH = venous pH + 0.04.
   3. Urine electrolytes: Get Na, K, Cr, osms. Get serum Cr and serum osms at same time. Diuretics must have been held for at least 6 h.
      a. Urine Na < 9 is consistent with dehydration (hanging onto salt).
      b. Urine Na > 20 but low serum Na and normal osms might be SIADH or renal failure.
      c. Urine anion gap: Useful in hyperchloremic metabolic acidosis. Measure the urine sodium + urine potassium - urine chloride. The remainder is ammonium ion.
         1) **Positive urine anion gap:** Implies renal wasting of bicarb.

     2) **Negative urine anion gap:** Implies GI wasting of bicarb.

B. Electrolyte abnormalities:

  1. Acidosis:

    a. Causes of anion gap acidosis:

      1) **Increased production of acid:**

        a) **Lactate.**

        b) **Ketosis:** DM, alcohol, starvation.

        c) **Ingestion:** Salicylates, methanol, ethylene glycol.

      2) **Decreased excretion of acid:** renal failure.

    b. Causes of non-anion gap acidosis: GI loss e.g. diarrhea, dilutional acidosis, carbonic anhydrase inhibitors, renal tubular acidosis,....

    c. Rx: Treat cause. Respiratory acidosis usually requires intubation. For severe acidosis, pH < 7.2, consider 44-88 mEq Na bicarbonate IV, in IV solution appropriate to the patient's fluid status. Don't correct to pH > 7.2.

      1) **Complications of bicarbonate rx:** Fluid overload, precipitation of acute tetany in patients with renal failure, and "relative CSF acidosis" (which can cause coma).

  2. Metabolic alkalosis:

    a. Causes: Vomiting, NG suction, dehydration, low K, loop diuretics, mineralocorticoids, compensation for chronic respiratory acidosis,....

    b. Rx: Alkalosis usually resolves with volume correction and KCl – careful with the latter in renal failure. Correct alkalosis promptly in patients with neuromuscular hyperexcitability or myocardial irritability.

  3. High sodium:

    a. H&P: Confusion, thirst, signs of dehydration.

    b. Rx: Correct Na slowly, to avoid brain edema, CHF. See Dehydration, p. 160.

  4. Low sodium:

    a. H&P: Confusion, seizures, signs of dehydration.

    b. Rx: Correct Na slowly, to avoid central pontine myelinolysis. See p. 160 for correction algorithms.

  5. SIADH:

    a. Criteria: Hyponatremia from inappropriately concentrated urine, without renal or adrenal dysfunction.

    b. DDx of SIADH: Dehydration, overhydration, renal failure, adrenal failure, hypothyroidism, cerebral salt wasting.

HYPERNATREMIA

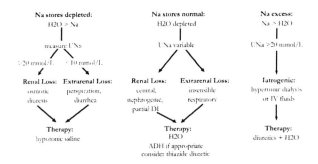

HYPONATREMIA

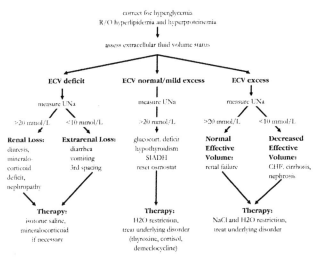

Figure 24. Diagnosis and treatment of hyper- and hyponatremia. UNa, urine Na; ECV, extracellular volume.

c. Causes of SIADH:
1) **Intracranial processes:** e.g. trauma, infection, tumor. However, you must rule out cerebral salt wasting—see below.
2) **Lung processes:** e.g. trauma, infection, tumor.
3) **Other:** Drugs, e.g. carbamazepine; malignancies, anemia, stress, acute intermittent porphyria.

d. Rx of SIADH:
1) **Acute:** IV NS, no free water. Furosemide if necessary.
2) **Chronic:** Fluid restriction; high-salt diet. Consider furosemide, demeclocycline 300 mg bid-qid.

6. **Cerebral salt wasting (CSW):** Hyponatremia from inappropriate excretion of salt in the kidney, via an unknown central mechanism. Unlike SIADH, patients with CSW are usually hypovolemic. Physical
exam, central venous pressure, pulmonary wedge pressure, plasma and
urine osms, etc. can help tell if the patient is hypovolemic. CSW is not
uncommon in SAH, and inappropriate fluid restriction for supposed
SIADH can worsen SAH vasospasm.

C. **Dehydration:**
  1. **H&P:** HR, SBP, urine output. Pt. is orthostatic if SBP drops > 15 mm
     Hg, or HR increases > 20 beats per minute from lying to sitting after 2
     min. Look at skin turgor, mucosal hydration.
  2. **Labs:** Electrolytes, BUN, glucose, osms, urinalysis.
     a. **Specific gravity:** < 1.015 suggests renal concentration defect, >
        1.030 = moderate dehydration, > 1.035 = severe.
     b. **Units:** in the following, Na is always measured in mEq/L.
  3. **Rx of dehydration:**
     a. **Discontinue diuretics.**
     b. **Replacement rate** = (deficit/time desired to replete) + mainte-
        nance rate.
        1) **Calculate deficit:**
           a) **Total deficit** = (old wt. - new wt.) <u>or</u> = 0.35(old wt.)(1 - old
              Hct/new Hct). Third-spacing will make these two numbers
              different; use the Hct estimate.
           b) **Free water deficit** (in hypernatremia) = $TBW(Na-140)/140$,
              where TBW = total body water = 0.5(wt.) for women,
              0.6(wt.) for men.
        2) **Calculate maintenance rate:** Per kg body weight.
           a) **For 1st 10 kg:** 4 ml/h/kg.
           b) **For 2nd 10 kg:** 2 ml/h/kg.
           c) **Above that:** 1 ml/h/kg.
     c. **Type of fluid to use:**
        1) **For Na 130-150** (isotonic dehydration): Replete with hypotonic
           dextrose solution (30-55 mEq Na/L); give 50% of replacement
           in 1st 8 hr; rest during next 16 h.
        2) **For Na < 130** (hypotonic dehydration): Replete with isotonic
           Na.
           a) **Beware central pontine myelinolysis**, which may result
              from over-rapid correction of hyponatremia. It presents as
              mutism, oculobulbar palsies, and quadriparesis. Correct Na
              slowly, not more than 1 U/h.
           b) **Beware seizures** when Na < 120.
        3) **For Na > 150** (hypertonic dehydration): Replete with D5 1/2
           NS.
           a) **Beware cerebral edema:** Correct Na slowly; shouldn't fall
              > 10 mEq/24 h.
  4. **Low potassium:**
     a. **H&P:** EKG changes (see p. 172), arrhythmia, muscle twitching,
        weakness.
     b. **Causes:** Vomiting, diarrhea, diuretics, alkalosis (intracellular K
        shift), hyperaldosteronism, familial periodic paralysis,....

    c. **Complicating conditions:** It is important to keep serum K > 4.0 in cardiac patients, asthmatics on β_2 agonists, and type II diabetics.

    d. **Rx:** Be cautious if there is renal failure. With normal patients, KCl 40 mEq PO q4h x 3 doses is usually enough. IV K correction should usually not exceed 10 mEq/h (note 40 mEq KCl/L at 100 ml/h is 4 mEq KCl/h)

5. **High potassium:**
   a. **H&P:** EKG changes (see p. 172), arrhythmia, flaccid paralysis.
   b. **Causes:** Acidosis, diuretics, renal failure, hemolysis, rhabdomyolysis, Addison's dz, familial periodic paralysis,....
   c. **Rx:** Stop K supplements. For serum K > 5.5 in renal failure, give sodium polystyrene sulfonate (Kayexalate) 30-60 g PO or enema. For emergent rx, consider 1 amp CaCl or Ca gluconate IV, or 2 amps Na bicarbonate with 2 amps D50 given with 10 U regular insulin IV.

6. **Low calcium:**
   a. **H&P:** Confusion, papilledema. Ca < 7 can cause tetany, laryngospasm, and seizures.
   b. **Correction for low albumin:** For every 1 g/dl albumin deficit, lower limit of normal Ca will decrease 0.8 mg/dl. Can also check ionized Ca, which is not influenced by protein, on an ABG. It is normally > 1.0.
   c. **Rx:** Ca carbonate 500 mg PO tid, or Ca gluconate 1-2 amps IV in 250 ml NS, given over 2-4 h. Beware giving Ca to patients on digoxin.

7. **High calcium:** Consider medicine consult.
   a. **H&P:** Abdominal pain, nausea, confusion, muscle weakness.
   b. **Causes:** Cancer, endocrine disorders, granulomatous dzs, renal failure,....
   c. **Rx:** Emergent if Ca > 15. Aggressive hydration, then diuretics; specific drugs such as pamidronate.

8. **Low magnesium:**
   a. **H&P:** Nausea, tremor, fasciculations, tetany.
   b. **Rx:** MgCl$_2$ 10 ml PO x 3 days; or MgSO$_4$ 2g IV in 250 ml D5 W IV. Be careful in renal failure.

9. **Low phosphate:** Treat with PO phosphate 2 tabs tid x 3 days, or Na- or K-phosphate 10 mmole over 6-8 h IV. Be careful in renal failure.

10. **High phosphate:** Treat with Phoslo 1-2 tabs PO tid.

GLANDS

A. Adrenal

1. **Adrenal insufficiency**
   a. **Neurological complications of adrenal insufficiency:** Lethargy, abdominal pain, neurological signs of low sodium (tremor, aphasia, ataxia, seizures, corticospinal tract signs) and high potassium. All male pts. with Addison's dz should be tested for X-linked adrenoleukodystrophy (see p. 113).
   b. **Adrenal crisis is an emergency:** Besides the above sx, see volume depletion and high BUN. Look for precipitants, e.g. infection,

MI.
- c. **Tests:**
    1) **Cortisol:** May be a better screen for adrenal suppression after prolonged steroid use. Best to do 8 am cortisol (normal 6-18 μg/dl), but in an emergency, draw a random level before giving steroids.
    2) **ACTH stimulation test:** Can be done on dexamethasone. Give ACTH (Cortrosyn) 0.25 mg IV; measure cortisol then and 60 min later. Normal is > 7 μg/dl increase, or total level > 18 μg/dl.
- d. **Rx:** Immediate hydrocortisone 100 mg IV q8h.

2. **Adrenal excess (Cushing's syndrome) or exogenous steroids:**
   - a. **H&P:** See p. 138 for signs of corticosteroid excess.
   - b. **Tests:**
       1) **Baseline 8 am cortisol:** Normal is 6-18 μg/dl.
       2) **Low-dose suppression:** Give dexamethasone 1 mg PO at 11 PM, draw serum cortisol at 8 AM. Cortisol < 5 μg/dl is normal, 5-10 is indeterminate, and >10 evidence for Cushing's syndrome.
       3) **High-dose suppression:** Helps tell pituitary ACTH hypersecretion from adrenal tumor or ectopic ACTH secretion. Give dexamethasone 8 mg PO at 11 pm, draw cortisol at 8 am. In 95% of pituitary ACTH hypersecretion, but not other causes, cortisol will decrease to < 50% of baseline. Phenytoin may interfere with this.

B. **Diabetes insipidus (DI):** Low antidiuretic hormone (ADH) causes dilute urine, water craving, danger of severely high Na.
   1. **Causes:** Pituitary damage, e.g. from surgery, head trauma, transtentorial herniation, neurosarcoid, A-comm aneurysm.
   2. **DDx:** Psychogenic polydipsia, osmotic diuresis, nephrogenic DI.
   3. **Tests:** If there is high clinical suspicion, the following four criteria are usually sufficient:
       - a. **Urine osms:** 50-150 mOsm/L or specific gravity < 1.005.
       - b. **Urine output:** > 250 ml/h (or > 3 ml/kg/hr).
       - c. **Serum sodium:** normal or high.
       - d. **Normal adrenal function:** The kidney needs mineralocorticoids to make free water, so steroids may unmask DI by correcting adrenal insufficiency.
   4. **Rx:** Intranasal desmopressin 10-40 μg bid (typically 20 μg); titrate to urine output.
       - a. **Post-op transsphenoidal surgery:** First try to keep up with fluid loss by IV or PO fluids, as desmopressin sometimes overtreats. Then try desmopressin in above dose range, although you will need to give it SQ or IV until nasal packs are removed.

C. **Diabetes mellitus:**
   1. **Neurological complications of DM:** Glucose-related mental status changes, neuropathy (see p. 72), increased stroke risk.
       - a. **Hypoglycemia:**
           1) **H&P:** Decreased POs or increased DM medications, with variable tremulousness, fatigue, dysarthria, confusion, seizures

(glucose usually < 30 mg/dl), coma with pupillary dilation and extensor posturing (glucose usually < 10).

2) **Tests:** Fingerstick glucose.

3) **Rx:** Emergent correction of glucose. Hypoglycemic coma can cause permanent neurological damage.

   b. **Diabetic ketoacidosis:**

1) **H&P:** Often type 1 diabetic with precipitating illness. See subacute polyuria followed by anorexia, confusion (glucose > 425 mg/dl), coma (glucose > 600).

2) **Tests:** Glucose, anion gap, ketones, osmolarity, ABG.

3) **Rx:** Correction of glucose, dehydration, potassium. Central pontine myelinolysis can occur when blood osmolarity is lowered more rapidly than brain osmolarity.

   c. **Nonketotic hyperglycemic coma:**

1) **H&P:** Often type 2 diabetic with infection. Steroids or phenytoin can sometimes be precipitants. Slower onset than DKA. Cerebral dysfunction and seizures are common.

2) **Tests:** Glucose, osmolarity, ABG.

3) **Rx:** First priority is maintaining blood pressure and cardiac output with IV fluid; correct glucose as needed.

2. **Regular insulin (CZI) sliding scale:** See Admission orders, p. 12. All diabetics should be covered with an insulin sliding scale while in house, even if they take only oral hypoglycemics at home. It is best to stop oral agents while pt. is in hospital, as glucose levels will vary from home levels.

3. **To convert regular (CZI) to NPH insulin:** NPH = (2/3)x(CZI used qd); give 2/3 of that in am, 1/3 in pm.

4. **Insulin preparations:**

Preparation	Onset	Peak	Duration (h)
Regular (CZI)	IV: immediate	15-30 min	2 h
	IM: 5-30 min	30-60 min	2-4 h
	SQ: 30-60 min	3-6 h	6-10 h
NPH	SQ: 3 h	8-12 h	18-24 h
Lente	SQ: 3 h	8-12 h	18-24 h
Protamine	SQ: 4 h	14-20 h	24-36 h
Ultralente	SQ: 4 h	16-18 h	30-36 h

Table 37. Insulin kinetics.

D. **Thyroid:**

1. **Neurological complications of hyperthyroidism:** Tremor, seizures, brisk reflexes, ophthalmopathy, proximal myopathy.

2. **Neurological complications of hypothyroidism:** Apathy, "hung-up" reflexes, myopathy, and high CPK. The slow muscle relaxation differs from myotonia in being more painful, and worse with exercise. Sometimes see seizures, obstructive sleep apnea, ataxia, hearing loss. T_3 may be better than T_4 for treating neurological complications.

3. **Tests:** First test TSH. If low, also check T_3 (triiodothyronine), T_4 (thyroxine), free T_4, and possibly antithyroid antibodies. If high, check

T_4.

E. Parathyroid: Psychiatric sx. Hyperparathyroidism can cause myopathy; hypoparathyroidism can cause seizures and other signs of low calcium and magnesium.

GUT

A. Abdominal pain
   1. **Common causes:** Infection, obstruction, ulcer, GI bleed, cholecystitis, pancreatitis, mesenteric ischemia, kidney stone, drug, toxin, urinary tract infection, ectopic pregnancy, ovarian torsion, inferior MI, herpes zoster.
   2. **H&P:** N/V, stool appearance, bowel sounds, rebound.
   3. **Tests:** Consider CBC, electrolytes, β-HCG, LFTs, amylase, UA, guaiac, abdominal X-ray, renal, right upper quadrant, or pelvic US, endoscopy, CT.

B. Constipation drugs: Never give anything from above if patient may be obstructed, i.e., lower "afterload" before raising "preload" or "inotropy."
   1. **Afterload reducers:** Dulcolax suppositories, Fleet's enemas, mineral oil enemas.
   2. **Preload:** Milk of magnesia 30 ml PO qid prn.
   3. **Inotropy:** Senekot 1-2 tabs bid prn, or Mg citrate 1 bottle, or lactulose 30 ml q2h until patient stools.
   4. **Stool softeners:** Colace 100 mg tid (not prn).

C. Diarrhea: Consider *Clostridium difficile* infection. Symptomatic rx: Lomotil 2 tabs PO qid prn, loperamide 2 mg PO prn (max 16 qd).

D. GI bleed (GIB)
   1. **Causes:**
      a. **Upper GIB:** Ulcer, varix, Mallory-Weiss tear.
      b. **Lower GIB:** Ischemia, thrombosis, intussiception, dysentery, colitis, diverticulosis, cancer, polyp, hemorrhoids, anal fissure/ulcer, AVM, angiodysplasia.
   2. **Nasogastric tube:** Cold lavage helps both dx and rx.
      a. **Contraindications:** Variceal bleeding.
      b. **False negatives:** Can have upper GIB with negative nasogastric lavage if bleed is duodenal. Look for high BUN.
   3. **Labs:** CBC, blood bank sample, PT, PTT, DIC screen, consider emergent endoscopy.
   4. **Rx of GIB:**
      a. **Orders:** NPO, orthostatic BPs, two large IVs, guaiac all stools, cardiac monitor. GI consult.
      b. **IV fluid or blood.**
      c. **Upper GIB:** IV ranitidine; consider *Helicobacter pylori* Abx. Ranitidine will increase phenytoin and warfarin levels.
      d. **Varices:** Consider pitressin + nitroglycerine, or octreitide (fewer side effects than vasopressin), or DDAVP (selective splanchnic bed constriction, emergent endoscopy for banding or sclerotherapy. Pt. should eventually be on longterm β-blockade.
      e. **Catastrophic bleed:** Blakemore tube.
      f. **Bleed on anticoagulants:** Reverse anticoagulation. See p. 127.

E. Hiccups: Consider brainstem lesion. Sometimes helped by baclofen 5 mg tid or chlorpromazine 25 mg bid.

F. Liver dz:

   1. Hepatic encephalopathy:

      a. H&P: Confusion, asterixis in pt. with liver failure, usually with precipitating illness.

      b. DDx: Wernicke's syndrome.

      c. Tests: Ammonia high, but it may take several days for patient to recover even after ammonia has returned to baseline. MRI may show T1 signal in basal ganglia, but is not that helpful. EEG will show slowing or triphasic waves.

      d. Rx: Lactulose, low-protein diet, oral neomycin.

   2. Bilirubin: Direct = conjugated. High indirect suggests hemolysis, ineffective erythropoesis, Gilbert's syndrome.

   3. Alkaline phosphatase up but 5'-nucleotidase normal suggests extrahepatic source of alk phos, e.g. bone.

   4. Transferases: ALT = SGPT; AST = SGOT.

	Direct/total bilirubin	Alk phos	Transferases
Hemolysis	+/++	nl	nl
Acute hepatitis	+/+	< 3x	SGOT > SGPT, > 400
Chronic hepatitis	+/+	< 3x	SGPT > SGOT, < 300
Acute cholestasis			T's often > alk phos
Chronic cholestasis	+/+	> 4x	< 300
Metastasis	nl	> 4x	< 300
Shock liver			SGPT >> SGOT

Table 38. Enzyme changes in liver disease.

G. Vomiting

   1. H&P: Nausea, color of vomit, diarrhea, fever, precipitating factors, diet, drugs, previous bowel surgery, vertigo, double vision, dysarthria, hearing loss. Neurological and abdominal exam. <u>Always</u> see the patient walk, to rule out ataxia.

   2. DDx: GI infection, vertigo (see p. 98), drugs, toxins, alcohol, obstruction, gastroparesis, perforated bowel, pregnancy, metabolic disturbance, e.g. uremia and hyperglycemia, brainstem lesion, severe fear or pain.

   3. Complications: Dehydration and orthostasis, acidosis, low K, gastric or esophageal (Mallory-Weiss) bleed, perforated esophagus.

   4. Tests: Electrolytes; consider tox screen, MRI for brainstem lesion.

      a. Abdominal X-ray is low-yield unless abdomen is severely tender or there is a high suspicion of obstruction.

   5. Rx of vomiting:

      a. Orders: NS + 20 KCl, NG tube, NPO.

      b. Anti-dopaminergic drugs (see p. 135).

         1) **Indications:** GI causes, surgery, radiation or chemotherapy.

         2) **Contraindications:** vertigo, tardive dyskinesia. In young people, watch for acute dystonia (see p. 60).

         3) **Butyrophenones:** e.g. droperidol 0.0625-2.5 mg q3-6h IV/IM. Sedating. Good for nausea from morphine.

4) **Phenothiazines:** Promethazine (Phenergan) 25-50 mg q4-6h PO/IM/PR has less risk of dystonia and seizures than prochlorperazine (Compazine). Contraindications include head trauma, epilepsy (lowers seizure threshold), tardive dyskinesia,....

5) **Metoclopramide** (Reglan): 10 mg IV/IM q2-3h or 10-30 mg PO qid before meals and qhs. A motility agent. Good for gastroparesis from autonomic neuropathy. Avoid in GI obstruction.

c. **Antihistamines:** e.g. meclizine (Antivert) 25 mg PO qid. Suppresses the vestibular apparatus in vertigo.

d. **Anticholinergics:** (q. v., p. 134). e.g. scopolamine.
   1) **Indications:** Motion sickness.
   2) **Contraindications:** Outlet obstruction, diabetic gastroparesis, glaucoma.

e. **Central:** e.g. granisetron (Kytril) 750 μg IV qd or 1 mg PO bid.

HEART

A. Cardiac code calls:

1. **What you need:** Call code team; bag-valve ventilator, 12-lead EKG; cardiac and oxygen monitor; large-bore IV access; stat blood gas, electrolytes, and CBC; defibrillator and code cart. Arrange for an ICU bed.

2. **Basic Life Support:** For all cases, two initial breaths, then compressions 80-100/min.
   a. **One rescuer:** 15:2 ratio of compressions to ventilations.
   b. **Two rescuers or pediatric:** 5:1 ratio of compressions to ventilations.

3. **Advanced Cardiac Life Support:**

BRADYCARDIA ACLS PROTOCOLS

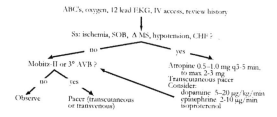

TACHYCARDIA ACLS PROTOCOLS

ABC's, oxygen, 12 lead EKG, IV access, review history
IF UNSTABLE: synchronous cardioversion (see below. R/o sinus tachycardia)
Cardioversion seldom needed for HR<150

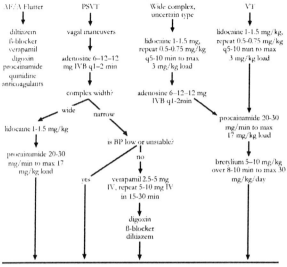

SYNCHRONIZED CARDIOVERSION
Consider paging cardiac anesthesia ; have suction and intubation kit ready
If awake, sedate with diazepam, midazolam, barbiturates with or without opiates
VT/AF: 100J, 200J, 300J, 360J
PSVT/A Flutter: 50J, 100J, 200J, 300J, 360J
polymorphic VT: treat as VF 200J, 300J, 360J

VF/PULSELESS VT SECOND LINE AGENTS

Lidocaine: 1.5 mg/kg (avg dose 100 mg) IVB, repeat in 3-5 min to max 3 mg/kg load

Bretylium: 5 mg/kg (avg dose 300-350 mg) IVB, repeat 10 mg/kg q5 min to max 30-35 mg/kg load

MgSO4 : 1-2 g IV, especially consider if patient in Torsade, known hypoMg or in refractory VF

Procainamide : infuse 30 mg/min to max 17 mg/kg load (avg dose 1-1.2 g)

NaHCO3 : 1 mEq/kg, consider if pt hyperkalemic, TCA OD, ? long arrest

Escalating or high dose epi: 1 then 3 then 5 mg 3-5 min apart or 0.1 mg/kg (avg dose 5-10 mg) q3-5 min

PULSELESS ACLS PROTOCOLS

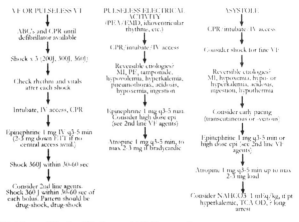

Figure 25. Advanced Cardiac Life Support (ACLS) protocols.

B. Neurological complications of heart dz: Embolic stroke, global hypoxia. MIs are risk factors for stroke, and vice versa. Atrial fibrillation, mechanical valves, and LV thrombus are all indications for anticoagulation to prevent stroke.

C. Arrhythmia
 1. **See also:** p. 170.
 2. **H&P:** Is pt. symptomatic during arrhythmia? What drugs is pt. on? Frequency, duration; what triggers and stops rhythm?
 3. **Tests:** EKG (compare with <u>old</u>), electrolytes, Ca, Mg, TSH, ABG, drug levels, CXR.
 4. **Atrial fibrillation:**
    a. **Causes:** Ischemia, PE, thyroid, drugs, conduction system problem, alcohol binge, post heart surgery.
    b. **EKG:** Absent P waves. If QRS is wide, consider V tach.
    c. **Rx of new A fib:** Consider cardiology consult. Unstable patients may require immediate cardioversion.
       1) **Rate control:**
          a) **Diltiazem:** Bolus 20 mg IV over 2 min; may repeat in 15 min. Consider verapamil or β–blockers.
          b) **Digoxin:** 0.5 mg IV, then 0.25 mg PO q8 x 2, then 0.125-0.25 mg qd. Not always the first-line agent these days. See Digoxin, p. 134.
          c) **Contraindications to A fib drugs:**
             • **Wide QRS complex** may actually be V tach, in which Ca channel blockers may be lethal. Consider adenosine. Treat like V tach: 75 mg lidocaine, cardiovert.
             • **Hypotension.**

- **Planning to DC cardiovert:** Digoxin may make cardioversion dangerous.
  2) **DC cardioversion:** Emergent if A fib has caused angina, hypotension, CHF.
  3) **Anticoagulation:** See p. 126.
5. **AV block:**
   a. **1st degree** = long PR. Don't treat unless bradycardic. Consider digoxin toxicity as cause.
   b. **2nd degree**
      1) **Mobitz I** (Wenckebach): Above bundle of His.
         a) **EKG:** gradual PR lenthening, narrow QRS, RR gradually shorter.
         b) **Rx:** Usually benign. If pt. is symptomatic, or if there is BBB, give atropine or pace.
      2) **Mobitz II:** Usually below His. May go to complete heart block.
         a) **EKG:** PR constant; usually wide QRS; occasional nonconducted P wave.
         b) **Rx:** Cardiology consult. Needs pacer even if pt. is asymptomatic. In the mean time, if symptomatic, use atropine, isoproterenol, or external pacing.
   c. **3rd degree:** Complete heart block. Treat as Mobitz II, but more urgently.
6. **Bradycardia:** See Cardiac code calls, p. 166.
7. **Junctional rhythm:**
   a. **EKG:** Narrow QRS but no Ps.
   b. **Rx:** Treat underlying condition (ischemia, dig toxicity). Treat paroxysmal junctional tachycardia like SVT, but carotid massage is less effective.
8. **Premature beats:** (PACs, PVCs). Usually treat only if pt. is symptomatic, but check with a cardiologist—some PVCs are "malignant."
9. **Supraventricular tachycardia (SVT, AKA PSVT):**
   a. **DDx:** V tach; rapid A fib, sinus tachycardia.
   b. **EKG:** Narrow-complex tachycardia always preceded by P waves. Tachycardia can cause ST depression and T-wave inversion, without ischemia, even after tachycardia has resolved.
   c. **Rx:** See Cardiac code calls, p. 166. Consult cardiology.
      1) **Adenosine:** If narrow-complex tachycardia.
         a) **Dosing:** Run rhythm strip; give 6-12-12 mg rapid bolus through peripheral IV (3-6-6 if central line) q1-2min.
         b) **Complications:** Watch for bronchospasm and low BP. If pt. is on theophylline, adenosine may not work.
         c) **Specific conditions:** OK to use in Wolff-Parkinson-White syndrome (WPW). In A fib/flutter, adenosine will uncover a string of nonconducted P waves.
      2) **Cardioversion:** If pt. has angina, hypotension, or CHF.
      3) **Carotid sinus massage** ± Valsalva maneuver. Need IV access and EKG monitoring. Rule out bruits first. Massage carotids only one side at a time: 10 sec on R; if no response, then 10 sec on L. This may convert A flutter to A fib.
      4) **Nodal blockers:**

   a) **Contraindications:** Avoid in wide-complex tachycardia, hypotension.
   b) **Verapamil** 5-10 mg IV over 2-3 min.
   c) **β-block:** Propranolol 0.15 mg/kg at 1 mg/min, or esmolol if h/o asthma.
   d) **Digoxin:** 0.5-0.75 mg IV/PO, then 0.25 mg q2h as needed.
10. **Torsades de pointes:**
   a. **Causes:** Things that lengthen QT interval, e.g. bradycardia, antiarrhythmics; phenothiazines, low K, Mg, or Ca; cerebral hemorrhage, ischemia, cardiomyopathy, congenital long QT, erythromycin + seldane.
   b. **EKG:** QRS amplitude varies sinusoidally, HR 160-180. Long QTc.
   c. **Rx:** Consult cardiology. Stop offending drugs. Give magnesium. Treat drug or metabolic imbalance. Consider lidocaine, phenytoin, isoproterenol (cautious if CAD), overdrive pacing.
11. **Ventricular fibrillation:** Call a code. See p. 166.
12. **Ventricular tachycardia:**
   a. **DDx:** Aberrantly conducted SVT (15%, usually with RBBB), tachycardic A fib. When in doubt, treat as V tach.
   b. **Causes:** Ischemia, MI recovery (especially with post-MI aneurysm), cardiomyopathy, prolonged QT, mitral valve prolapse, drug toxicity, metabolic disturbance.
   c. **EKG:** > 6 wide QRSs at 100-200 bpm. ST and T changes in direction opposite to major QRS deflection. LAD (compared with axis in sinus). AV dissociation. Monophasic or biphasic RBBB QRSs with LAD and R/S < 1 in V6.
   d. **Rx:**
      1) **Sustained V tach:** Call a code. See p. 166.
      2) **Nonsustained V tach:** Consult cardiology immediately. Treat V tach if pt. is symptomatic during V tach, or if runs are increasing in frequency or length (this suggests impending V fib).
13. **Varying rhythm:**
   a. **Identical Ps:** Suggest sinus arrhythmia; observe.
   b. **Changing Ps:** Suggest wandering atrial pacemaker or multifocal atrial tachycardia.
      1) **Causes:** COPD, hypoxia, digoxin toxicity, mitral regurgitation, myocardial scar.
      2) **Rx:** Correct hypoxia, electrolytes; try verapamil or diltiazem, β-block (not if COPD), consider Ia antiarrhymics, amiodarone. Avoid digoxin.
   c. **No P waves:** Suggests A fib.
D. **Electrocardiogram**
   1. <u>**Compare all EKGs with old ones.**</u>
   2. **Heart rate:** Normally 60-100. One box = 0.04 sec.
   3. **Rhythm:** Look at both Ps and QRSs. If there is arrhythmia (see p.168), ask
      a. **What is relation between P and QRS?** Ps best seen in leads II and V1. Should be upright there.
      b. **Wide or narrow QRS?**
      c. **QRS regular or irregular?**

4. **Intervals:**
   a. **PR:** 3-5 boxes. < 0.12 sec suggests WPW; > 0.2 = AV block.
   b. **QRS:** > 3 boxes (0.12) suggests ventricular arrhythmia or BBB. Look in widest QRS, usually V1, V5.
   c. **QT:** 7-10 boxes (0.28-0.40 sec) for normal rate.
      1) **QTc** = QT/(RR interval)$^{1/2}$. Less than 0.42 for men, 0.43 women.
      2) **DDx:** Drugs (quinidine, procainamide, TCAs, phenothiazines), hypothermia, electrolyte abnormality, pentamidine, idiopathic.

5. **Axis:** Normal if upright in I, F (or, more liberally, if -30 to +90).

6. **P waves:** Leads II and V1 show Ps best.
   a. **Absent Ps:** Atrial fibrillation (see p. 168).
   b. **Inverted Ps** in II, III, or F: low atrial or junctional pacemaker.

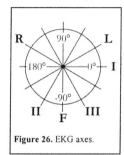

Figure 26. EKG axes.

7. **QRS waves:**
   a. **Q wave** = Significant when more than 1 box wide or deep, or more than 1/3 of the following R wave. Normal in III, or small isolated Q in I, L, F, V4-V6. Q in III can also suggest PE.
   b. **Poor R-wave progression (PRWP):** DDx = Anterior MI, LBBB.
   c. **Too-good RWP** (i.e. R in V1-V2 larger than in V3): posterior MI, RV infarct, lateral MI, RBBB, RV hypertrophy, WPW syndrome.
   d. **LV hypertrophy:** S in V1 + R in V5 > 35 mm. LAD, wide QRS, and T slants down slowly and returns rapidly.

8. **ST segments:** Compare voltages with TP segment, not PR.
   a. **ST elevation:** Normal < 1 mm limb leads; < 2 mm chest.
      1) **DDx** = Acute MI, LBBB, J point elevation (concave, upsloping ST in young people).
      2) **Persistent ST elevations:** DDx = persistent ischemia, LV aneurysm, pericarditis (concave, widespread, especially anterior).
   b. **ST depression:** DDx = ischemia, digoxin (upsloping), exercise, strain, PE (especially lead II).

9. **T waves:** Can be down in III, L, F, V1-V2. Brain injury can cause non-specific T-wave changes, but this is a diagnosis of exclusion.
   a. **Peaked (hyperacute) T waves:** Ischemia, high K. T's should be <5 mm in limb leads; <10 mm in chest leads.
   b. **T-wave flattening:** Ischemia, post-MI, low K.
   c. **T-wave inversion (TWI):** Ischemia, post-MI, BBB (should be in opposite direction), strain (biphasic and asymmetric in V5-V6), sometimes just from tachycardia. Normally inverted in R.
   d. **Pseudonormalized Ts:** i.e. formerly inverted, now flat or upright. Suggests ischemia.
   e. **T-wave axis:** Should be <50 from QRS axis.

10. **U waves:** Low K, low Mg.

E. **Miscellaneous EKG syndromes:**

1. **β-blockers:** bradycardia, AV block.

2. **Bundle branch block (BBB):** if QRS > 0.12. Left BBBs can have fixed ST elevations not associated with MI, but always worry if the elevations change.

3. **Calcium:**
   a. **Calcium channel blockers:** Sinus arrest, AV block.
   b. **High Ca:** Short QT, tachycardia.
   c. **Low Ca:** Long QTc.

4. **Digoxin toxicity:** Upsloping ST depressions, tachycardia, AV block, junctional rhythms, bradycardic junctional escape, V tach, V fib.

5. **Potassium:**
   a. **High K:** In sequence as K rises, see peaked T (esp V_2-V_4), ST depression, decreased R waves, PR lengthening, flat P, wide QRS, long QT, torsades.
   b. **Low K:** Flattened T, U wave, ST depression, PSVT, A fib, long QT.

6. **Pulmonary embolus:** Often nonspecific sinus tachycardia, sometimes SI-QIII-TIII (big S in I, Q and TWI in III), right axis deviation and right BBB.

F. **Coronary artery dz:**
   1. **Acute MI:**
      a. **DDx of chest pain:** Aortic dissection, peri- or myocarditis, PE, PTX, perforated ulcer, cholecystitis, pancreatitis, rupture of the esophagus, musculoskeletal pain.
      b. **Tests:** See Suspected MI protocol, below.
      c. **Rx:** Emergency cardiology or medicine consult.
         1) **Reduce cardiac work:**
            a) **But beware low BP** in carotid dz, renovascular dz, aortic stenosis, RV infarct, big anterior MI, tamponade.
            b) **Nitroglycerine:** SL and IV to increase coronary perfusion.
            c) **β-blocker:** IV metoprolol, then PO metoprolol or inderal.
               • **Loading metoprolol:** 5 mg IVP over 2 min x 3 doses to lower heart rate, while SBP > 100, HR > 50, PR < 0.24. Then 50 bid, and titrate up, with hold parameters as above.
               • **Beware PO BP drugs** that can't reverse fast.
               • **Use cautiously** in COPD, CHF, inferoposterior or big anterior MI.
            d) **Morphine:** To reduce pain and preload, 2-5 mg IV. Watch BP.
         2) **Treat clot:** Chew aspirin, IV heparin ; consider lysis, angioplasty, bypass.
            a) **Heparin:** For unstable angina, ST depressions, or chest pain with a baseline BBB.
            b) **Consider thrombolysis:** For ST elevations. <u>Absolute contraindications</u> = recent surgery, stroke, GI or brain bleed.

   2. **Complications of MI:**
      a. **Arrhythmias.** Cardiac monitor.
      b. **Hypotension.** Suspect RV infarct in anyone with hypotension during an inferoposterior MI.

   c. **Congestive heart failure:** See below.

3. **Chest pain orders:** Check vitals, EKG during pain, nitroglycerine SL q5min x 3 if SBP > 90, O_2 2 L/min, call resident, post-pain EKG. Consider Mylanta, morphine.

4. **Suspected MI protocol:**
   a. **Cardiology consult.**
   b. **Drugs:** Aspirin, heparin SC or IV (for unstable angina, needs several days of heparin to cool off), O_2, IV access, Colace, sucralfate, nitropaste q4h (see Admission orders, p. 12, for doses; adjust if carotid dz or long-standing HTN).
   c. **Labs:** CPK q8min x 3, profile 7, PTT (bid if IV heparin), Ca/Mg/phos, CBC, LFTs, lipids, drug levels, EKG q am x 3; consider echocardiogram, ETT with thallium (make pt. NPO after midnight) or persantine-thallium scan (no caffeine or theophylline before scan).
   d. **Orders:** Bedrest with bedside commode, check orthostatic BP, guaiac stools, I/Os, daily weights, low-salt and low-cholesterol diet, cardiac monitor (pt. may travel without), old chart to floor quickly.

G. **Preoperative cardiac evaluation:** If pt. has any of the following CAD markers, consider pre-op cardiology consult: age > 70, prior angina or MI, prior CHF or ventricular arrhythmia, diabetes, positive stress test.

H. **Congestive heart failure:**
   1. **Systolic failure:**
      a. **H&P:** Ask about SOB, precipitants, cardiac history. Check rales, jugular venous pressure, edema.
      b. **DDx:** Lung dz, noncardiac edema.
      c. **Rx:** Goal = decreased preload.
         1) **Acute:** Sit pt. up with legs dangling. Oxygen, morphine 2-5 mg IV, nigroglycerine SL or IV, furosemide 40 mg IV.
         2) **Severe:** Consider digoxin, CPAP (helps LV pump, but bad if preload is low), dobutamine, intubation.
         3) **Orders:**
            a) **R/O MI orders.**
            b) **I/Os:** Fluid restrict, low salt, daily weights, ± bladder catheter.
            c) **Labs:** Digoxin level, repeat K and CXR after diuretics, consider echocardiogram.
            d) **Drugs:** Digoxin, furosemide, captopril (or isosorbide dinitrate + hydralazine).
      d. **Diastolic dysfunction:**
         1) **Rx:** Goal is maintained preload, decreased afterload, and decreased contractility. Nitrates and diuretics are OK acutely, but try verapamil long-term.

I. **Blood pressure:**
   1. **Hypertension:**
      a. **Causes:** MI, stroke, cerebral bleed, drug withdrawal or overdose, renal, endocrine, anxiety, aortic dissection or coarct, ecclampsia.
      b. **Hypertensive crisis:** Usually DBP > 130 or SBP > 250. Need evidence of other end-organ damage: heart, brain, renal. Check fundi.

      1) **Rx:** Arterial line + IV nitroprusside or labetalol. See p. 136.

        a) **Contraindications to nipride:** Cerebral edema or coronary ischemia.

        b) **Avoid** SL nifedipine, which can drop BP too fast.

      2) **Time course:** Decrease BP <u>gradually</u>, by 25% in the following intervals:

        a) **If cerebral hemorrhage,** in 6-12 h.

        b) **If papilledema,** in 3-6 h.

        c) **If CHF, LV failure, dissection,** in 15 min.

    c. **Antihypertensive drugs:** For PO control, see p. 123. Consider nifedipine 10 mg SL (danger of hypotension), or metoprolol 50 mg PO. For IV blood pressure control, see p. 136.

      1) **Aortic aneurysm:** Use labetolol (lowers HR as well as BP) unless there is CHF.

      2) **CHF:** Use ACE-I, diuretics, α_1 blockers. Avoid β–blockers, diltiazem, verapamil.

      3) **CAD:** Use β–blockers, Ca channel blockers, ACE-I. Avoid diuretics, hydralazine.

      4) **Cerebral bleed or stroke:** Use β-blockers, then α–blockers, then ACE-I.

      5) **COPD:** Use Ca blockers, ACE-I, diuretics. Avoid β-blockers.

      6) **Diabetes:** Use ACE-I, α_1 blockers, Ca blockers. Avoid β-blockers, diuretics.

      7) **Diastolic dysfunction:** Use β–blockers or Ca blockers.

      8) **Heart block or bradycardia:** Avoid β-blockers, verapamil.

      9) **Hyperlipidemia:** Use α–1 blockers, Ca blockers. Avoid β–blockers, diuretics except indapamide.

      10)**Peripheral vascular dz:** Use Ca blockers, ACE-I, diuretics. Avoid β–blockers.

      11)**Renal failure:** Use loop diuretics, Ca blockers, ACE-I (especially for DM or nephrotic syndrome, but use very cautiously). Avoid β–blockers, K-sparing diuretics.

      12)**Sexual dysfunction:** Use ACE-I, Ca blockers. Avoid β–blockers, central α–blockers, diuretics.

2. Hypotension:

    a. **Causes:** Heart rate, pump, or volume problem, drug effect, blood loss, dehydration, sepsis, third-spacing, adrenal insufficiency, tension PTX.

    b. **Tests:** EKG, ABG, orthostatic BP, electrolytes, CBC, cultures, CXR.

    c. **Rx:**

      1) **Trendelenberg position:** Head of bed down 10 degrees. Of short-term benefit only; increases risk of aspiration.

      2) **If bradycardic:** Correct rate before administering fluid or pressor.

      3) **Normal saline IV:** Be careful if CHF.

      4) **Hold offending drugs.**

      5) **Blood:** For volume (be careful if CHF).

6) **Oxygen:** Especially if anemic (be careful if COPD, because of risk of CO_2 retention).
7) **Take cultures:** If febrile.
8) **Pressors.** Mild hypotension may benefit from midodrine 10 mg PO tid. For IV pressors see p. 136.

J. Pulmonary artery catheter: (Swann-Ganz catheter).
 1. **Alternatives:** Green dye cardiac output (requires arterial line and central line); echocardiography, a better physical exam,....
 2. **Indications:** Note there is no evidence that Swanns improve outcome. They may worsen it. They are useful for telling cause of shock (e.g. septic vs. cardiogenic); cause of pulmonary edema (e.g. cardiogenic vs. increased permeability); monitoring the effects of fluids, inotropes, pressors, afterload agents, and vasodilators, and optimizing oxygen transport.
 3. **Relative contraindications:** Coagulopathy, thrombocytopenia, endocardial pacemaker, severe pulmonary hypertension, ventricular arrhythmias, LBBB (have external pacer ready in case of complete heart block), prosthetic right heart valve.
 4. **Complications:** Include these risks on the consent form.
    a. **During puncture:** Arterial puncture, pneumo- or hemothorax, air embolism, nerve injury, thrombosis.
    b. **During advancement of catheter:** Arrhythmias, cardiac perforation and tamponade, BBB.
    c. **During maintenance of catheter:** Pulmonary artery rupture, mural thrombus, infection, valve damage, pulmonary infarction.
 5. **Normal values**
    a. **CVP:** Central venous pressure, 5-8 mm Hg.
    b. **RA:** Right atrial pressure, 0-8 mm Hg.
    c. **RV:** Right ventricular pressure, (15-30)/(0-4) mm Hg.
    d. **PA:** Pulmonary artery pressure, (15-30)/(6-12) mm Hg.
    e. **PCWP:** Pulmonary capillary wedge pressure, 1-10 mm Hg.
    f. **LVP:** Left ventricular pressure, (100-140)/(3-12) mm Hg.
    g. **CO:** Cardiac output, 4-8 L/min (= HR x stroke volume).
    h. **CI:** Cardiac index, 2.5-4.2 $L/min/m^2$.
    i. **SVR:** Systemic vascular resistance, 770-1500 $dynes/sec/cm^5$.
    j. **PVR:** Pulmonary vascular resistance, 20-120 $dynes/sec/cm^5$.
    k. **MAP:** Mean arterial pressure, 70-105 mm Hg = (1/3)(SBP-DBP) + DBP.

K. Cholesterol emboli syndrome
 1. **Causes:** Often after arterial catheterization, vascular surgery.
 2. **Sx:** Necrotic foot lesions, conjunctival petechiae, renal failure, depression and dementia, nausea, and anorexia.
 3. **Rx:** Symptomatic.

INFECTIONS

A. See also: CNS infections, p. 45.

B. Fever workup

   1. **H&P:** Vital signs, pain, cough, shortness of breath, dysuria, diarrhea, new drugs. Lung, cardiac, abdomen, mouth, skin, fundi, pelvic exams. Inspect line sites and wounds.

   2. **Tests:** CBC, urinalysis, urine culture; consider CXR, sputum culture, stool culture, wound culture, line tip culture throat swab, LP, shunt tap, ascites tap, induced sputum for TB, HIV test, echocardiogram,.... Drug fever and tumor fever are diagnoses of exclusion only.

      a. **Blood cultures:** If temperature > 101.5° F. If pt. has a central line, draw one off each port, and one peripherally.

      b. **LP:** If neurological signs, severe HA, meningismus, recent brain trauma or surgery. See lumbar puncture, p. 191; cerebrospinal fluid, p. 17.

   3. **Rx:**

      a. **Remove foreign bodies:** Change central lines, consider removal of bladder catheter, ventricular shunt,....

      b. **Empiric Abx:** Always check for penicillin allergies. Except in cases where Abx must be given immediately, make sure all relevant cultures have been taken before starting Abx. Not every patient with a fever needs Abx.

      c. **Control fever:** e.g. with acetaminophen; consider cooling blanket. Fever can worsen infarct size, strain the heart, and cause dehydration.

      d. **Fever and neutropenia:** If absolute neutrophil count (WBC x %PMNs) < 500, order neutropenic precautions, nystatin swish and swallow 10 ml qid; consider bleeding precautions if platelets < 20.

C. Human immunodeficiency virus (HIV): See also neurological consequences of HIV, p. 46.

   1. **Protease inhibitors:** Crixivan = indinavir, Invirase = saquinavir, Norvir = ritonavir, Viracept = nelfinavir.

   2. **Other antiretrovirals:** Epivir = 3TC, Rescriptor = delavirdine, Retrovir = AZT, Videx = DDI, Zerit = D4T.

   3. **Secondary infections:** Bacterial, *Pneumocystis carinii*, toxoplasmosis, fungal, mycobacterial, viral (PML, CMV, HSV, VZV), syphilis,....

      a. **Prophylactic Abx:** Under certain CD4 counts, pts. should get azithromycin for *Mycobacterium avium,* Bactrim for *P. carinii* and toxoplasmosis, fluconazole for fungi.

   4. **Secondary neoplasms:** Kaposi's sarcoma; lymphoma.

D. Abx and antivirals:

   1. **Neurological side effects of:**

      a. **Acyclovir:** May see encephalopathy in association with renal failure, methotrexate, or interferon.

      b. **Aminoglycosides:** Vestibular and ototoxicity, neuromuscular blockade (especially in myasthenia).

      c. **Amphotericin B:** Rare headache, tremor, confusion, akinetic mutism.

    d. Isoniazid: Seizures, altered mental status, optic neuritis.

    e. Metronidazole: Distal axonopathy, psychosis, hallucinations.

    f. Penicillin derivatives: Rare myoclonus, asterixis, coma.

    g. Tetracyclines: Rare pseudotumor cerebri in infants.

    h. Vancomycin: Ototoxicity.

    i. Zidovudine (AZT): Headache, insomnia, sometimes confusion, seizures, myopathy.

E. Empiric antibiotic recommendations for adults: Review Abx when culture data become available. These guidelines do not take into account all details that may apply to any given patient.

SYNDROME	FIRST CHOICE	ALTERNATE
Community-acquired pneumonia		
GS unhelpful or suggests h. Flu or M. catarrh.	Cefuroxime or ceftriaxone IV ± macrolide	Levofloxacin PO/IV
GS suggests *S. Pneumoniae*	Penicillin IV	Cefuroxime or ceftriaxone
GS suggests *S. Aureus*	Nafcillin	Cefazolin
Aspiration likely	Penicillin IV ± metronidazole	Clindamycin IV
Underlying dz (COPD, CHF, DM, etc.)	Cefuroxime ± erythro	Erythro + TMP-SMX
Known/suspected HIV+	TMP-SMX ± erythro	
Hospital acquired pneumonia		
Non-intubated	Ceftriaxone ± gent	Clindamycin + gent
Intubated	Gent + (ticarcillin or cefazolin)	Ceftriaxone + gent
P. aerguinosa	Ceftazidime + gent	Ticarcillin + gent
Sepsis syndrome or suspected bacteremia		
Intraabdominal/pelvic source	Amp + metronidazole + gent	Amp/sulbactam + gent
Urinary source suspected	Amp ± gent	Vanco + gent
Unknown source	Gent + metronidazole + (nafcillin or vanco)	Vanco+ ceftriaxone + metronidazole
Neutropenic host with fever	Ceftazidime	Gent + (ticarcillin or ceftazidime)
Ear, nose, throat		
Acute otitis or sinusitis	Amoxicillin	TMP-SMX
Dental infection	Penicillin or clindamycin	Penicillin + metronidazole
Acute bacterial meningitis - see p. 47 (adult) or p. 111 (pediatric)		
Urinary tract infection		
All pts. requiring Abx	Amp + gent	TMP-SMX or levofloxacin
Skin & soft tissue infection		
No underlying dz	Nafcillin or cefazolin	Erythromycin or ceftriaxone
Underlying dz (DM, vascular insufficiency, IVDA)	Ticarcillin/clavulanate or amp/sulbactam	(Ceftriaxone or vanco) + (gent or levofloxacin)

Table 39. Empiric antibiotics. Amp = ampicillin, erythro = erythromycin, gent = gentamycin, GS = gram stain, TMP-SMX = trimethoprim-sulfamethoxazole, vanco = vancomycin.

BACTERIA	Pen	Oxa	Cphl	Van	Cln	Ery	Tet	Chlr	T-S	Ntr[1]
Staph aureus	12	76[2]	76	100	78	60	94	–	94	100
Coag-neg Staph.	18	47	47	100	68	40	86	–	63	100
Staph saprophy.	40	–	77	100	92	45	88	–	92	100
Pneumococci	73	–	–	100	–	87	86	92	72	–
α streptococci	70	–	79	100	92	55	73	–	79	–
β strep (A,G)	100	–	100	100	96	84	82	–	88	–
β strep (B)	97	–	100	100	100	87	16	–	0	–
Enteroccoci	80	–	–	84[3]	–	–	36	97	–	89

Table 40. Gram positive susceptibilities (% susceptible). Pen, penicilllin; Oxa, oxacillin; Cphl, cephalothin; Ery, erythromycin; Tet, tetracycline; Chr, chloramphenicol; Cln, clindamycin; Van, vancomycin; T-S, trimethoprim/sulfamethoxazole; Ntr, nitrofurantoin [1] urine isolates only. [2,3] All pts with oxacillin (methicillin) resistant Staph. aureus (MRSA) or vancomycin-resistant Enterococci (VRE) should be on CONTACT PRECAUTIONS.

BACTERIA	Amp	Tic	Cfz	Cftx	Cftz	Azt	Imi	Gen	Ami	Levo	T-S
Citrobacter diversus	0	0	91	100	–	100	100	100	100	100	98
Citrobacter freundii	2	76	17	75	–	84	100	93	100	82	79
Enterobacter aerogenes	0	80	23	95	–	90	100	100	100	100	99
Enterobacter cloacae	0	79	5	90	–	86	99	96	100	93	91
Escherichia coli	70	71	94	99	–	100	100	98	100	99	86
Haemophilus influenzae	75	–	–	100	–	–	–	–	–	–	74
Klebsiella spp.	0	4	83	94	–	96	100	95	100	94	90
Proteus mirabilis	92	95	97	100	–	100	100	96	100	95	93
Proteus vulgaris	0	96	0	100	–	100	100	96	100	95	93
Pseudomonas aeruginosa	–	88	–	–	98	85	94	94	97	78	–
Serratia marcescens	0	84	0	100	–	99	100	98	100	92	97

Table 41. Gram negative susceptibilities (% susceptible). Amp, ampicillin; Tic, ticarcillin; Cfz, cefazolin; Cftx, cefotaxime; Cftz, ceftazidime; Azt, aztreonam; Imi, imipenem; Gen, gentamicin; Ami, amikacin; Chlr, chloramphenicol; Levo, levofloxacin; T-S, trimethoprim-sulfamethoxazole.

Table 42. Commonly Used Antibiotics.

Antibiotic	NORMAL DOSE	ADJUSTED MAX. DOSE IN RENAL FAILURE			DIALYSIS REMOVES?
		GFR >50	GFR 10-50	GFR <10	
Gentamicin	80 mg IV q8h	1.0-1.7 mg/kg q(8 x serum creatinine) h			Yes (H, P)
Tobramycin	80 mg IV q8h	1.0-1.7 mg/kg q(8 x serum creatinine) h			Yes (H, P)
Amikacin	300 mg IV q8h	5 mg/kg q(8 x serum creatinine) h			Yes (H, P)[2]
Cefazolin	1 g IV q8h	q8h	bid	qd	Yes (H), no (P)
Cefotaxime	1 g IV q6h	NC	NC	1-2 g bid	Yes (H), no (P)
Cefotetan	1 g IV q12h	NC	1-2 g qd	1 g qd	Yes (H)
Ceftazidime	1 g IV q8h	NC	1-2 g bid	1 g qd	Yes (H, P)
Ceftriaxone	1 g IV q24h	NC	NC	NC	No (H)
Cefuroxime	0.75 g IV q6h	NC	0.75-1.5 g q8h	0.75 g qd	Yes (H, P)
Cephalexin	0.5 g PO bid	NC	NC	0.25-0.5 g qd	Yes (H, P)
Cephalothin	0.5 g PO qid	NC	NC	NC	Yes (H, P)
	1 g IV q4h	1-2 g q6h	1-2 g q6h	1 g q8h	Yes (H, P)
Amoxicillin	0.5 g PO tid	NC	0.25-0.5 g bid	0.25 g bid	Yes (H), no (P)
Amox-clavulanate[3]	0.5 g PO tid	NC	0.25-0.5 g bid	0.25 g bid	Yes (H), no (P)
Ampicillin	1 g IV q4h	NC	1-2 g q8h	1-2 g bid	Yes (H), no (P)
	3 g IV q6h	NC	1.5-3 g bid	1.5-3 g qd	
Ampi-sulbactam[4]	0.5 g PO qid	NC	NC	NC	No (H, P)
Dicloxacillin	0.5 g IV q6h	NC	0.25-0.5 g q8-12h	0.25-0.5 g bid	Yes (H)
Imipenem-cilastatin[5]	4 g IV q4-6h	NC	2-3 g q6h	2-3 g bid	Yes (H), no (P)
Mezlocillin	1.5 g IV q4h	NC	NC	NC	No (H, P)
Nafcillin	1.5 g IV q4h	NC	NC	NC	No (H, P)
Oxacillin	2 MU IV q4h	NC	NC	1-2 MU q4h	Yes (H), no (P)
Penicillin G	0.5 g PO qid	NC	NC	NC	Yes (H), no (P)
Penicillin VK					

Drug	Dose					Dialysis (H, P)
Piperacillin	4 g IV q6h	NC	NC	2-4 g q8h	2-4 g bid	Yes (H), no (P)
Piper-tazobactam[6]	4.5 g IV q6h	NC	NC	2.25 g q6h	2.25 g q8h	Yes (H)
Ticarcillin	3 g IV q4h	NC	NC	2-3 g q6h	2 g bid	Yes (H, P)
Ticar-clavulanate[7]	3.1 g IV q6h	NC	NC	3.1 g q6-8h	2 g bid	Yes (H)
Ciprofloxacin	0.5 g PO bid / 0.4 g IV q12h	NC	NC	0.25-0.5 g bid	0.25-0.5 g qd	
Levofloxacin	0.5 g PO/IV qd	NC	NC	0.4 g q12-18h	0.4 g q18-24h	
Ofloxacin	0.4 g PO/IV bid	NC	NC	0.4 g q24h	0.2 g q24h	
Azithromycin	0.5 g qd	Unknown	Unknown	Unknown	Unknown	No (H, P)
Clarithromycin	0.5 g PO bid	Unknown	Unknown	Unknown	Unknown	No (H, P)
Erythromycin	1 g IV q6h / 0.5 g PO q6h	NC	NC	NC	NC	No (H, P)
Clindamycin	0.6 g IV q8h / 0.3 g PO qid	NC	NC	NC	NC	No (H, P)
Tetracycline	0.5 g PO qid	0.5 g q8-12h	NC	Avoid	Avoid	No (H, P)
Doxycycline	100 mg PO/IV q12h	NC	NC	NC	NC	No (H, P)
Aztreonam	1 g IV q8h	NC	NC	NC	1 g IV bid	Yes (H, P)
Chloramphenicol	1 g IV/PO q6h	NC	NC	NC	NC	Yes (H), no (P)
Metronidazole	0.5 g IV/PO q6h	NC	NC	NC	NC	Yes (H), no (P)
Nitrofurantoin	50-100 mg PO q6h	NC	NC	Avoid	Avoid	Yes (H)
TMP-SMX[8]	DS PO bid / 160/800 mg IV q6h	NC	NC	2-5 mg/kg bid	Avoid	Yes (H), no (P)
Vancomycin	0.5 g IV q6h	1 g q1-3d	NC	Follow blood levels; redose when <10	NC	No (H, P)
	0.125 g PO q6h	NC	NC	NC	NC	Not absorbed

GFR, glomerular filtration rate; H, hemodialysis; P, peritoneal dialysis; NC, no change; MU, million units.

1,2: Following an initial loading dose, therapeutic levels can be maintained by administering (1) 1 or (2) 3.5 mg/kg IV after each hemodialysis OR by adding (1) 4 mg/L or (2) 20 mg/L to the peritoneal dialysis fluid

3,5: Dosage refers to active component only, e.g. (3) amoxicillin and (5) imipenem, respectively (each 250 and 500 mg tablet of amoxicillin-clavulanate contains 125 mg clavulanate; imipenem/cilastatin is premixed 1:1).

4,6,7: Dosage refers to total dose of antibiotic and inhibitor, e.g. ampicillin/sulbactam = 2:1, ticarcillin/clavulanate = 3 0.1, and piperacillin/tazobactam = 3:0.375.

8: Dosage is based on TMP component/kg; SS tab = 1 amp IV = 80 mg TMP/400 mg SMX, DS tab = 160 mg TMP/800 mg SMX; oral liquid suspension = 40 mg TMP/200 mg SMX per 5 mL).

KIDNEYS

A. **H&P:** Fluid intake, drugs (include NSAIDS), urine output, pain. Cardiac exam, kidney tenderness, palpable bladder, edema.

B. **Neurological complications of kidney failure:**
  1. **Uremic encephalopathy:**
     a. **H&P:** Renal dz ± precipitating illness, with obtundation or agitation, myoclonus, generalized seizures in 30%.
     b. **DDx:** Malignant hypertension, dialysis disequilibrium syndrome, stroke.
     c. **Rx:** Treat renal failure. If you use phenytoin for seizures, take account of renal failure's effects on phenytoin levels (see p. 129). Although phenobarbital is excreted by kidneys, it is also useful for seizures, since levels are unaffected by uremia.
  2. **Dialysis disequilibrium syndrome:** Acutely during or after dialysis, with headache, muscle cramps, confusion, seizures, or coma. Probably caused by cerebral edema.
  3. **Dialysis dementia syndrome:** Subacute memory loss, personality change, apraxia, dysarthria, myoclonus, seizures (EEG shows bursts of slowing and spikes).

C. **Hematuria workup:** Stop anticoagulants, change bladder catheter and consider irrigation, consider renal ultrasound, cystoscopy, antineutrophil cytoplasmic Ab (ANCA), antiglomerular basement membrane antibody.

D. **Causes of acute renal failure:**
  1. **Prerenal:** Hypovolemia or hypotension from dehydration, sepsis, bleed, or heart failure; liver failure.
  2. **Renal:** Acute tubular necrosis (ATN) (from ischemia, toxins, radiocontrast agents, hemo- or myoglobinuria), glomerulonephritis, DIC with cortical necrosis, arterial or venous obstruction, acute tubulointerstitial nephritis (drug reaction, pyelonephritis, papillary necrosis, intrarenal precipitation (calcium, urates, myeloma protein).
  3. **Postrenal:** Obstruction from prostatism, tumor, or stones.

E. **Tests:**
  1. **Blood:** BUN, creatinine, serum electrolytes, Ca/Mg/phos, CBC. Check CPK if there could be rhabdomyolysis.
  2. **Urine:** Urinalysis, sediment, culture, urine eosinophils, urine electrolytes after 6 h off diuretics.
  3. **FENa:** Fractional excretion of sodium. Nonspecific in nonoliguric acute tubular necrosis.
     a. **FENa** = $100 \times (UNa \times SCr)/(SNa \times UCr)$, all in mg/dl.
     b. **Causes of low FENa:** Dehydration, Na-avid renal failure, cirrhosis, nephrotic syndrome, CHF, glomerulonephritis, oliguric contrast-induced renal failure.
     c. **Causes of high FENa:** Recent diuretics; renal failure.

	Prerenal	ATN
BUN	Up	Up
Serum Cr	~nl	Up
BUN/S Cr	>20	nl (13-20)
Urine Na	<20	>40
U Cr/S Cr	>40	<20
Urine osms	>500	<350
FeNa	<1	>2
IV fluid helps?	Yes	No

Table 43. Prerenal kidney failure vs. acute tubular necrosis.

  4. 24h urine: For protein and creatinine in chronic renal failure.
    a. Creatinine clearance = [urine Cr (mg/dl)][vol (ml)]/{[serum Cr (mg/dl)][time (min)]}
    b. Estimated creatinine clearance: (inaccurate if Cr changing).
      1) **Male** = (140 - age)(wt in kg)/(72 x serum Cr in mg/dl)
      2) **Female** = 0.85 x male.
  5. Other tests: Consider renal ultrasound, renal scan, glomerulonephritis workup.
F. Orders: Renal diet (60 g protein, 2 g Na, K) unless on dialysis, when need protein supplements. Strict I/O, bladder catheter, daily weights.
  1. Stop nephrotoxins: gentamycin, ACE-I, NSAIDS; renally dose cimetidine, Abx.
  2. NSAIDS: Can lower Na, increase K, cause proteinuria, acute interstitial nephritis.
  3. Gentamycin: Worsens renal failure. However, pts. on dialysis can have gentamycin; redose after each dialysis.
  4. IV fluids: If dehydrated.
  5. Diuretics: If oliguric. Furosemide IV; consider adding chlorothiazide or mannitol. Follow I/Os q1h. Hold diuretics if pt. has no response, or furosemide level will build up and cause ototoxicity.
  6. Chronic renal failure: Nephrocaps 1 qd, Amphogel 30 ml qid (avoid Mg compounds), Phoslo (calcium acetate) 1-2 tabs. Consider erythropoeitin, iron, calcium, vit D, bicarb (600-1200 mg PO bid).

LUNGS

A. Blood gases
  1. A-a gradient: Lowered by diffusion defects, R-L shunt (doesn't correct on 100% O_2), V/Q mismatch. Fi = fraction of inspired gas, PA = alveolar partial pressure, Pa = arterial partial pressure, RQ = respiratory quotient.
    a. A-a = PAO_2 - PaO_2 = nl 3-16 mm Hg.
      1) **Age correction:** should be < 2.5 + 0.25x(age). If pt. < 30 yr, A-a gradient should be < 8 mm Hg.
    b. PAO_2 = (FiO_2)(barometric - water vapor pressure) - pCO_2/RQ
        = FiO_2(713) - pCO_2/0.8
      1) **On room air:** FiO_2(713) = 143; nl PAO_2 is 100 mm Hg.
      2) **On 100% ventilation:** PAO_2 should be 673 mm Hg. This doesn't apply to 100% oxygen by face mask.

   c. **PaO$_2$** > 70 gives full hemoglobin saturation.

   d. **FiO$_2$** increase of 10% adds 5 to PaO$_2$.

  2. **Respiratory effects on pH:** See also Electrolytes, p. 157.

   a. **High pH:** Suggests hyperventilation. Rule out CHF, PTX, PE.

   b. **Normal pH + high pCO$_2$:** Suggests chronic CO$_2$ retention.

   c. **Low pH:** Suggests acute hypoxia or sepsis.

B. Acute dyspnea or hypoxia

  1. **H&P:** Check VS, temperature, alertness, respiratory rate and pattern; listen to lungs, heart; assess jugular distension, ankle swelling; ask about pleuritic pain.

  2. **DDx:** Pulmonary edema (cardiac, vasogenic, neurogenic), COPD, MI, PE, PTX, effusion, upper airway obstruction, lung hemorrhage, hypoventilation from drugs or CNS problem, hyperventilation from acidosis or anxiety.

  3. **Tests:**

   a. **Blood gas:** On room air if possible. See above for interpretation. Hct performed on blood gas is sometimes inaccurate.

   b. **D-dimer:** Will be high in PE, but very nonspecific.

   c. **Portable CXR.**

   d. **EKG:** Look for ischemia;signs of PE (see below).

   e. **Lung scan:** Consider V/Q scan or Pagram plus possible IVC filter placement.

  4. **Rx:** "L-M-N-O-P," i.e. Lasix, Morphine, Nitrates, Oxygen, and Posture. Beware of causing hypotension, especially in patients with cerebrovascular dz.

   a. **IV diuretics:** For exacerbation of chronic CHF, but not for flash pulmonary edema.

   b. **Morphine:** For hyperventilation in pain and decreased preload in CHF. Beware of somnolence.

   c. **Nitrates:** For pulmonary edema and cardiac ischemia.

   d. **Oxygen:** Avoid causing CO$_2$ retention in COPD. Consider mechanical ventilation (see below).

   e. **Posture:** Have pt. sit up, with legs dangling.

   f. **Benzodiazepines:** For anxiety. They can help prevent breath stacking in COPD, but beware somnolence.

C. COPD flare

  1. **H&P:** Baseline FEV1 (See PFTs, below), functional limitations, number of pack-years smoking, home oxygen, previous intubations. Lung and heart exam.

  2. **DDx:** See acute dyspnea, above.

  3. **Tests:** ABG, CXR, EKG, K, Mg, CBC, theophylline level. Sputum for gram stain, culture. If suspect TB: PPD, sputum for AFB x 3. Consider sputum for cytology x 3.

  4. **Drugs:**

   a. **Albuterol:** Nebulizer 0.5 ml in 2.5 ml NS q2-4h. Ipratroprium inhaler 2 puffs qid or glycopyrrolate nebulizer 0.8 ml in 2.5 ml NS q8h, Use inhaler, not nebulizer if pt. intubated.

   b. **Methylprednisolone:** 60 mg IV q6h, then taper (eventually switch to inhaled steroids). Ranitidine or sucralfate while on steroids.

   c. **Empiric Abx:** See Infections, p.176.

    5. **Orders:** Guaiac stools if on steroids. Chest physical therapy. Check peak flow.

D. Lung mass workup: Chest CT through the adrenals; consider needle biopsy or bronchoscopy.

E. Pulmonary embolus (PE)

    1. **Risk factors:** Trauma, surgery, prior PE, bedrest, cancer, CHF, hypercoagulable states, oral contraceptives.

    2. **Prophylaxis:** (If not already anticoagulated). Heparin 5000 U SQ bid, or pneumoboots. If pt. has been in bed more than 24 h, check venous ultrasound before starting boots.

    3. **H&P:** Dyspnea, anxiety, tachycardia, pleuritic pain, cough.

    4. **DDx of PE:**

        a. **Small PE:** Pneumothorax, hyperventilation, asthma, MI, CHF, serositis.

        b. **Big PE:** RV infarct, tamponade, air embolism.

    5. **Labs:**

        a. **General:** ABG, D-dimer (useless if recent trauma or surgery), CXR.

        b. **EKG:** Often see only sinus tachycardia. See also Electrocardiogram, p. 170.

        c. **Venous ultrasounds (LENIs):** 97% sensitive for thrombus above the knee, 80% below. Not good for pelvic clots.

        d. **Ventilation-perfusion (V/Q) scan:** Consider going straight to pulmonary angiogram if high risk. V/Q scan may be useless if CXR is abnormal or there has been a previous PE.

        e. **Pulmonary angiogram:** Pulmonary HTN and renal failure are relative contraindications.

    6. **Rx of PE:**

        a. **Heparin:** (Unless contraindication, e.g. recent brain surgery), with bolus, for 5-7 d, then warfarin, or SQ heparin bid for 6 wk.

        b. **Thrombolyse:** If life-threatening PE.

        c. **Inferior vena cava filter:** For recurrent PE or pt. who can't be anticoagulated.

F. Pulmonary function tests: (PFTs)

Test	COPD	Restrictive	Neuromusc.
TLC (total lung capacity)	Up	Down	Normal
RV and FRC (residual volume, functional residual capacity)	Both up	Both down	Both normal
VC (vital capacity)	nl-down	Down	Down
FEV1 (forced exp. vol. in 1sec)	Down	nl or up	Normal
MIP and MEP (mean inspiratory and expiratory pressure)	Normal	Normal	Down

Table 44. Pulmonary function tests.

G. Stridor or laryngeal edema: See Allergy, p. 154.

H. Ventilators and oxygen delivery:

    1. **Nonendotracheal oxygen delivery systems:**

        a. **Passive ventilation:** Nasal cannula, face mask, or face tent, 100% non-rebreather.

    b. **Partially assisted ventilation:**

       1) **Continuous positive airway pressure (CPAP):** Indications: sleep apnea, or to keep alveoli open in COPD.

       2) **Biphasic positive airway pressure (BIPAP):** AKA intermittent positive pressure breathing. Indications: chronic neuromuscular dz; not great for COPD.

2. Endotracheal intubation: Call anesthesia, respiratory therapy.

    a. **Indications:** To maintain oxygenation or ventilation, protect airway or manage secretions, or to allow adequate sedation. Remember that intubation makes it hard to follow pt.'s neurological exam.

    b. **Anesthetics for intubation:** See p. 126 and 139. Most wear off fast—but neurological abnormalities may linger longer.

    c. **Stat CXR after intubation:** Endotrachial (ET) tube should be below the thoracic inlet, and > 2 cm above carina. Check CXR daily.

3. Ventilator setting orders: Specify FiO_2, TV, IMV, PEEP, PS, and type of oxygen monitoring (e.g. continuous saturation monitor).

    a. **Typical ventilator settings:**

       1) **Oxygen (FIO_2):** 40% (start at 100%).

       2) **Tidal volume (TV):** 600-800 ml (7-10 ml/kg). More if COPD, less if restrictive lung dz.

       3) **Respiratory rate (RR):** 8-12. Less if COPD, more if restrictive dz.

       4) **Positive end expiratory pressure (PEEP):** Start at 5.

       5) **Pressure support (PS):** 10-15. PS ~8 just overcomes resistance of ET tube.

4. Ventilator modes:

    a. **Intermittent mandatory ventilation (IMV, SIMV):** For patients without adequate spontaneous minute ventilation. Specify RR and TV. Can be used with backup pressure support for patient's spontaneous breaths.

    b. **Pressure support (PS, PSV):** For patients with adequate spontaneous respiratory drive. Specify PS only; adjust so that TV is 7-10 ml/kg. Ventilator has apnea alarm so pt. will get a backup IMV breath if necessary.

    c. **Pressure control (PC, PCV):** For severe COPD, adult respiratory distress syndrome. Set RR, inspiration pressure, and inspiration time. It is like PS, but maintains a minimum RR. Pt. usually needs sedation and paralysis to tolerate PC.

5. Changing ventilator settings: In some hospitals, only respiratory technicians are allowed to do so.

    a. **Ventilation increases** (and thus pCO_2 decreases) with increased PS, TV, RR.

    b. **Oxygenation increases** with increased PEEP, FiO_2, or inspiration time (unless there is a significant pulmonary or cardiac shunt).

       1) **To follow oxygenation across different FiO_2:** use pO_2/FiO_2 as index. Normal = $100/0.2 = 500$.

    c. **PEEP vs. PS:** PEEP is like CPAP, PEEP + PS is like BIPAP.

6. Ventilator complications:

    a. **Infection:** Most patients get colonized; don't treat presence of bacteria in sputum with Abx unless abundant PMNs in sputum, fever, high WBC, or copious secretions.

    b. Tracheal stenosis: Associated with prolonged intubation. Generally plan tracheostomy after 21 d.

    c. Oxygen toxicity: Try to keep FiO_2 below 50%.

    d. Gastric distension: From ET tube leak. Place NG tube.

    e. Blood pressure changes: Higher intrathoracic pressure lowers BP.

        1) **Intubation:** Treat with IV fluids—but remember to diurese pt. at extubation, to avoid fluid overload.

        2) **COPD:** Inadequate exhalation (breath stacking) causes auto-PEEP and may be helped by decreasing RR.

    f. Barotrauma: From high peak inspiratory pressure.

    g. Pneumothorax.

  7. Extubating:

    a. Criteria: Pt. on room air, PEEP (=CPAP) 5, no IMV, should have RR < 30, few secretions, PIP < 40, normal blood gas.

    b. Preparation: Empty stomach. HOB up 45 degrees. Tell the respiratory technician. Extubate to 100% O_2, continuous O_2 saturation monitor. Watch for laryngeal edema (see p.154).

  8. Tracheostomy wean: Consult anesthesia or surgery, speech pathology.

    a. Indications: Pt. can tolerate breathing off the ventilator, no need for frequent suctioning.

    b. Methylene blue test: Put dye in tube feeds to r/o aspiration

    c. Tracheostomy types: Usually pt.'s first tracheostomy is an 8 Portex, sutured. This may later change to a 4 cuffless Shiley with Passy-Muir valve. Consider a fenestrated tracheostomy.

    d. Button tracheostomy If pt. tolerates the above. If there is no need for suctioning, you may eventually decanulate.

PREGNANCY AND CHILDBIRTH

A. Neurological complications of pregnancy:

  1. Cerebral hemorrhage: The risk increases with each trimester.

    a. Causes: AVMs and aneurysms are most common; also DIC, anticoagulants, placental abruption, mycotic aneurysm, metastatic choriocarcinoma, and eclampsia.

    b. Rx: Hyperventilation, hypothermia, and steroids are safe; try to avoid mannitol. Surgery is based on same criteria as nonpregnant patients.

  2. Cerebral infarction: About 1 in 3000 pregnancies. 70% are arterial occlusion, 30% secondary to cerebral venous thrombosis.

  3. Cerebral venous thrombosis.

  4. Chorea gravidarum. Rare. Usually starts after first trimester, remits after delivery. See Choreoathetosis, p. 60, for DDx. Haloperidol is a relatively safe rx.

  5. Eclamptic encephalopathy: Associated with hypertension, proteinuria, edema, oliguria, hyperreflexia, and seizures. Usually young prima gravidas, > 20 wk gestation. Give magnesium 4 g IV over 15 min, then 1-2 g/h, along with Ringer's lactate. Seizures may also be treated with diazepam or phenytoin.

6. **Neuropathies of pregnancy:** Bell's palsy, carpal tunnel syndrome, and meralgia paresthetica are most common.
7. **Obstetrical palsies:** From compression by fetal head, forceps, or leg holders. Most common is L4-5 palsy, compressed by fetal brow as it crosses the pelvic rim.
8. **Pseudotumor cerebri:** Usually presents around wk 14 and spontaneously resolves in 1-3 mo.

B. **Effects of pregnancy on neurologic conditions:**
1. **Migraine:** Most migraineurs improve during pregnancy, but migraines may also start then, especially in the first trimester. Acetaminophen; barbiturates and low-dose opiates are the safest analgesics. Avoid serotonin agonists, ergots, and propranolol. Amitriptyline may be acceptable but should be stopped 2 wk before delivery.
2. **Multiple sclerosis:** Attacks are less likely during pregnancy, but more likely postpartum. Epidural anesthesia is not contraindicated by MS.
3. **Myasthenia:** Avoid magnesium sulfate, scopolamine, large amounts of procaine. Watch for neonatal myasthenia for 72 h. Myasthenia often flares postpartum.
4. **Neuropathy:** CIDP and Charcot-Marie-Tooth dz may worsen.
5. **Tumors:** Most enlarge during pregnancy and shrink somewhat afterwards. Increased ICP may be an indication for premature termination of the pregnancy. ICP generally does not increase during labor, however.
6. **Seizures:** Anticonvulsants may harm the fetus, but so may seizures. The rate of birth defects is as high as 10%. Give folate 1 mg qd, and keep anticonvulsant doses as low as possible. Monitor free levels, because plasma proteins change during pregnancy. If doses are increased in pregnancy, return them to initial levels postpartum to avoid toxicity. There is a 10-fold higher incidence of seizures within 24 h of delivery.

PROCEDURES

PROCEDURE NOTE

A. Should contain: Indication; consent; sterile preparation; anesthesia; findings; labs sent; pt.'s tolerance.

ARTERIAL BLOOD GAS

A. Need: ABG kit, optional xylocaine + TB needle, lab slips.

B. Procedure: Expel gas from syringe, extend wrist, iodine prep, inject xylocaine, have gauze within reach, feel pulse, bevel up, impale artery vertically, let syringe fill 1-2 ml. Expel any air bubbles, cap it, label it, put on ice if not sent immediately.

C. Results: Hct and K values vary from those done in a heparinized tube.

ARTERIAL LINE

A. Consent: Bleeding, infection, thrombosis, nerve damage.

B. Need: Mask, xylocaine and TB needle, 20 ga 1¼ inch angiocatheters, heparinized saline hookup or flush and plug, wire, sterile towels or small sheet, wrist board with padding to hyperextend wrist, thick adhesive tape, iodine, sterile 4x4 gauze 10-pack, sterile gloves, 3-0 suture.

C. Check for ulnar-radial anastomosis: Have pt. make a fist; press on radial artery, open hand. Whole hand should turn pink, not just ulnar side.

D. Setup: Tape wrist, slightly hyperextended, to board, perhaps to bed too. Prep arm, sterile drape, flush catheter tip with heparinized saline, put on gloves, anesthetize wrist, unwrap wire.

E. Stick: Impale artery bevel up, at 45 degrees, flatten angiocath somewhat. When blood spurts out, thread wire, remove needle, and advance catheter.

F. Secure: If flow looks good, remove wire, connect catheter to transducer; suture catheter, cover with clear plastic dressing.

G. Removal: Hard hand pressure for 5 min'; check for continued bleeding.

BLOOD DRAWS

A. Electrolytes: Green top (heparinized).

B. CBC, Blood bank: Lavender top (EDTA).

C. General chemistries: Red top (clotted).

D. PT/PTT: Blue top (citrate).

E. Glucose: Grey top (K oxalate).

F. Hypercoagulability panel: Usually four blue tops and a large red top.

CALORIC TESTING

A. Check ears: Tympanic membrane perforation is a contraindication. Wax can block test.

B. Tilt head: 30 degrees, so horizontal canal is perpendicular to floor.

C. Instill water: Use angiocatheter (with needle removed). Temperature should be 7° above and below body temperature; wait 5 min after each

test. In comatose patient consider using ice water. Normally start seeing nystagmus at end of infusion.
D. DDx:
1. **Brainstem damage:** Smaller or absent response on damaged side.
2. **Inner ear dz:** Smaller or absent response on damaged side.
3. **Cerebellar dz:** Fixation doesn't suppress nystagmus (normally does).
4. **Progressive supranuclear palsy:** Poor response with eyes closed, good if open.

CENTRAL VENOUS LINE

A. See also: Venous access, p. 193.
B. Indication: Pressors, nipride, nitroglycerine > 400 µg/min.
C. Check: PT, PTT before placing line.
D. Consent: Complications = bleeding, clot, infection, PTX, air embolus, nerve damage, arrythmia.
E. Need: Central line kit, 10 ml heparin 100 U/ml (not 1000), sterile gloves, sterile sponges, Betadine, suture, dressing. Consider replacement caps for all ports, sterile gown, sterile towels, mask.
F. Preparation: Clear space behind bed. Pt. in Trendelenberg to keep air bubbles from brain. Towel roll between shoulders. Tape open heparin flush bottle upside down to IV pole for easy sterile access. Iodine prep from ear to sternal notch for internal jugular; consider prepping subclavian region too. Open towels; use their drape to cover pt.'s abdomen. Open kit, extra gloves, sutures onto field. Drape patient sterilely, leaving enough room to identify landmarks. Then put on sterile gloves and gown. Remove cap from brown port, for wire to go through. Do not let line touch any nonsterile surface, of course. Place needles on syringes, line, suture, and extra gauze within reach. Xylocaine to skin. Then fill that syringe with heparin flush. Leave a few ml to suck air out of catheter.
G. Internal jugular: Safer than subclavian; easiest from right side.
1. **Find vein:** Use small needle. Anesthetize. Stand on R side of pt., feel carotid, aim with syringe on small needle through the triangle between the bellies of the sternocleidomastoid to the ipsilateral nipple. Aspirate as you go in until you hit IJ and blood. Slip syringe on larger needle (with catheter) next to the smaller one, while aspirating. Withdraw the smaller needle; withdraw larger syringe and needle from needle, thread wire down catheter. Always hold wire with one hand.
2. **Insert line:** Remove catheter from wire, cut down along wire with scalpel, insert and remove dilator. Thread line down over wire; at some time you will need to start pushing wire back up into line. Go about 15 cm. Remove wire. As wire passes brown port clamp, clamp it to avoid air embolus before you screw on cap. Use heparin syringe to suck air from each port and then flush port.
3. **Secure line:** Anesthetize and suture line, tying to inner holder only; then clip outer holder on (allows moving line without resuturing). Suture far end too. Cover with iodine gel, gauze, Tegaderm.
4. **Check line:** Stat CXR with wet read to check line placement (should be in inferior vena cava) and r/o PTX.
H. Subclavian: Easier than internal jugular; easiest from left side.

1. **Find vein:** Use medium needle. Find middle third (angle) of clavicle, start about 2 cm away, aim straight at lower edge with lidocaine needle; march down it, injecting and pulling back, until you are underneath. Insert the large needle, noting position of bevel (up). Hold needle with left hand, aspirate with right. Consider putting little finger in sternal notch as landmark. March the same way, aspirating with large needle, until you are under the clavicle; then rotate syringe so that you are parallel with clavicle and bevel is pointing down toward toes. Keep against clavicle, advance aspirating, until you are in vein. Remove syringe, thread wire.
2. **Insert and secure line:** Follow protocol as above for IJ. Go 17 cm for L subclavian.
3. **Taking line out:**
   a. **Need:** Suture removal kit, chuck, pt. in Trendelenberg position.
   b. **Procedure:** Pt. exhales slowly as you withdraw line.

LACERATIONS

A. **Need:** Saline, sterile bowl, kidney bowls to irrigate into, 60 ml luer lock, 20 ga angiocath, gauze, towels, chuck, 1% lidocaine, syringe + needle, sterile gloves, suture (for skin, 5-0 or 4-0 prolene; for scalp, galea, and muscle, Vicryl).

LUMBAR PUNCTURE

1. **Indications:** To rule out meningitis, hemorrhage; help diagnose carcinomatosis, demyelinating dz.
2. **Contraindications:**
   a. **Increased ICP from mass lesion:** Check for papilledema and retinal hemorrhages; CT for signs of mass effect (if there is high suspicion of meningitis, start Abx before CT or LP).
   b. **Coagulopathy:** 2 U fresh frozen plasma usually brings INR to < 1.5.
   c. **Infection over area to be punctured:** Never do an LP in a pt. with fever and back pain until you have ruled out empyema with MRI.
3. **Consent:** Headache (in 10%; see LP headache, p. 44), bleeding, infection, nerve damage.
4. **Need:** LP kit, gloves x 2, chuck, povidone, alcohol, extra black-topped tubes, extra lidocaine. Best to have a working IV before LP, in case you need to give mannitol.
5. **Position:**
   a. **Lying:** Fetal position; make sure hips are even.
   b. **Sitting:** Easier, but can't read opening pressure. Have pt. lean over a chair.
6. **Procedure:**
   a. **Locate L3-L4 interspace:** Parallel with superior iliac crest. Sterilize skin with iodine, don sterile gloves, drape, anesthetize skin, set up tubes and manometer.
   b. **Advance needle:** Slowly with bevel up and stylet in, parallel to bed and towards the navel. Withdraw stylet frequently to check for CSF flow.

      1) **Paresthesias:** If pt. feels tingling in a leg, angle needle away from that leg.

      2) **Difficult punctures:** Especially when the interspace is tight, or when landmarks are hard to palpate, it often helps to anesthetize a larger area and then make repeated parallel penetrations, marching up or down the spine, rather than angling the needle around within one penetration. If unsuccessful at L3-L4, try L4-L5 and L2-L3. Try it with the patient seated. If all fails, you can order a fluoroscopically guided LP .

  c. **When you get flow,** rotate needle so bevel points toward head, attach adaptor tube and then stopcock with manometer. Measure CSF pressure.

      1) **Opening pressure:** nl < 200 mm water.

      2) **If OP measurement is important:** Get pt. to straighten legs before you read it.

      3) **If OP > 400-500:** Danger of herniation. Put stylet back, leave needle in to prevent CSF leak. Take out only amount of CSF in manometer. Infuse dexamethasone 10 mg IV push, and 20% mannitol IV 0.25-0.5 g/kg over 20-30 min. Recheck pressure at end of infusion; need to get it below 400 before withdrawing needle.

  d. **After measuring OP:** Screw first white-topped tube onto bottom of manometer. Remove manometer. Change tubes when they are full. Having patient valsalva may speed flow.

  e. **When finished,** reinsert stylet, withdraw needle, clean off iodine. Lying down treats but does not prevent post-LP headache.

7. **Send specimens:** The following are possible tests—don't run all of them on everyone. Save extra CSF. For interpretation of results, see cerebrospinal fluid, p. 17.

  a. **Hematology:** Tubes 1 and 4 for cell count. (0.5 ml each).

  b. **Chemistry:** Glucose, protein, xanthochromia (0.5 ml).

      1) **Xanthochromia:** To spin it yourself, put 1 ml in centrifuge x 2 min; look at supernatant. (Don't bother if fluid is clear.)

  c. **Immunology:** Oligoclonal bands (> 2.5 ml).

  d. **Microbiology:** (> 3ml). Culture (bacterial ± fungal), VDRL (only if serum positive or if high suspicion), antigens (*H. influenzae,* strep-, meningo-, and cryptococcus), AFB stain (2.5 ml), Lyme titer. Cultures are useful if drawn < 2 h after starting empiric Abx.

  e. **Cytology:** (2-3 ml).

  f. **Others:** Lactate + pyruvate to rule out mitochondrial dzs. Covered, on ice. CSF for paraneoplastic Ab is usually <u>unnecessary:</u> serum levels are more sensitive.

NASOGASTRIC TUBE

A. **Indications:** Feeding (small tube, e.g. Enteroflex), to rule out GI bleed or protect lungs from vomiting (large tube, e.g. Salem sump).

B. **Contraindications:** Esophageal varices.

C. **Need:** Tube (NG tube or Enteroflex), large syringe with correct tip (Luer for Enteroflex, catheter tip for Salem sump), lubricating jelly, cup of water + straw, stethoscope, sterile saline if lavage, basin for aspirated contents, tape, benzoin, safety pin.

D. Insertion:
1. **Measure distance:** Between patient's nose and stomach to get idea of how far to advance it. Lubricate tip.
2. **Have pt. sit completely upright:** Head bent forward, with straw to water in mouth (if compliant).
3. **Push tube straight back:** While pt. swallows. Tube may curl in back of mouth; feel with finger. Beware of biters.
4. **To rule out GI bleed:** Aspirate contents and guaiac them (acidity of stomach contents sometimes causes false positive result), then lavage with ice-cold saline.

E. Checking placement:
1. **Cover extra holes in tube:** With your fingers. Blow air into gut and listen with stethoscope for bubbles.
2. **Securely tape tube:** To nose and pin it to pt.'s garment. Consider soft restraints in confused patients.
3. **If the tube is an enteroflex:** Get a CXR before pulling wire, to check for tube position and r/o PTX.

F. Drugs: If drugs must now go down NG tube, stop extended-release drugs, since they can't be ground. Write order to flush tube after all drugs. Sucralfate is a notorious tube-clogger.

VENOUS ACCESS

A. Peripheral IVs:
1. **Need:** Gloves, chuck, gauze, iodine/alcohol prep, lidocaine, tourniquet, angiocatheter, extension set or plug, saline flushes in 3-ml syringes, Tegaderm, tape.
2. **Placement:** Try for the forearm; antecubital IVs pinch off when the pt.'s arm moves. In pts. with poor arm veins, consider the feet and, occasionally, external jugular.

B. Percutaneously inserted central catheters (PICC lines):
1. **Indications:** For pt. who will need an IV more than 7 d, or who needs central delivery of drug. Especially good for home IV therapy. You should not draw blood samples off them.
2. **Placement:** often by specially trained PICC nurse. Difficult ones may be done fluoroscopically.

C. Central venous neck lines (IJ, SC):
1. **Indication:** Urgent central delivery of drugs, e.g. pressors, nipride, nitroglycerine > 400 μg/min, or frequent blood draws. Consider PICC as non-emergent alternative.
2. **Placement:** See Central venous lines, p. 190.

D. Quinton catheters: For dialysis, pheresis. Usually inserted by surgeons.

E. Hickman catheters: Surgically placed semi-long term (e.g. several months) central access, e.g. for chemotherapy. External ports on chest.

F. Portacaths: Surgically placed long term (e.g. years) central access, e.g. for chemotherapy. Has subcutaneous ports in chest.

G. Clogged catheters: Try urokinase: slowly instill 5,000 U.

INDEX

Notes

Notes

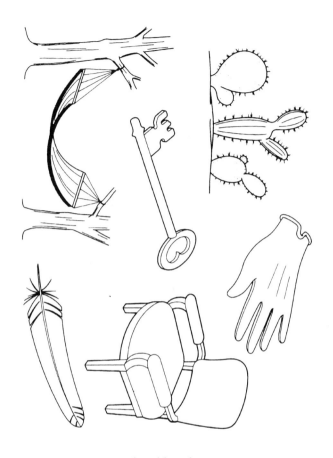

Baseball player.
I got home from work.
They heard him speak on the
radio yesterday evening.

Figure 27. Tests for anomia and alexia from the NIH stroke scale.

Notes